THE SECRETS AND EVOLVING TRENDS OF KOREAN LONGEVITY

THE SECRETS AND EVOLVING TRENDS OF KOREAN LONGEVITY

Edited by
Kwangsung Park · Jae-Young Han · Jeonghwa Lee · Sang Chul Park

Written by
Kwangsung Park · Jae-Young Han · Jeonghwa Lee · Minjeong An
Kyung A Cho · Jeong Gwan Cho · Hyong-Ho Cho · Min Jhon · Min-gu Kang
Sung Sun Kim · Ki-Hong Kim · Jonghwa Kim · Jeongjae Lee · Sungsu Lee
Kichae Min · Clara Yongjoo Park · Minho Shin · Kyung Chul Yoon · Sang Chul Park

First published November 2023
Publisher: Kwang-Seog Kim

https://doi.org/10.23228/9788968499906
ISBN: 978-89-6849-990-6 (93510)
Price: 20,000 Won

Published by Chonnam National University Press,
77 Yongbong-ro, Bukgu, Gwangju,
Republic of Korea, 61186
Tel: 82-62-530-0571～3, Fax: 82-62-530-0579

This study was supported by Chonnam National University (Grant number: 2023-1750-01) and Chonnam National University Hospital Biomedical Research Institute (BCRI23069)

The Secrets and Evolving Trends of

Korean Longevity

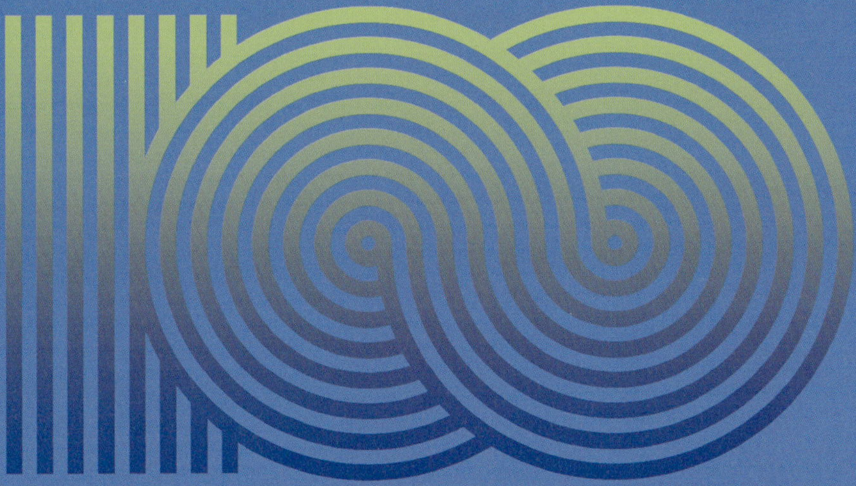

Edited by Kwangsung Park, Jae-Young Han, Jeonghwa Lee, Sang Chul Park

CHONNAM NATIONAL UNIVERSITY PRESS

Lists of Contributors

Minjeong An, PhD, RN, FNP-BC
Associate Professor, Chonnam National University College of Nursing,
Gwangju, Republic of Korea

Kyung A Cho, PhD
Professor, Department of Biochemistry, Chonnam National University Medical School,
Hwasun, Republic of Korea

Jeong Gwan Cho, MD, PhD
Emeritus Professor, Department of Cardiovascular Medicine,
Chonnam National University Medical School, Gwangju, Republic of Korea

Hyong-Ho Cho, MD, PhD
Professor, Department of Otolaryngology-Head and Neck Surgery,
Chonnam National University Medical School

Jae-Young Han, MD, PhD
Chairperson, Professor, Department of Physical and Rehabilitation Medicine,
Chonnam National University Hospital & Medical School, Gwangju, Republic of Korea

Min Jhon, MD
Department of Psychiatry, Chonnam National University Medical School,
Gwangju, Republic of Korea

Min-gu Kang, MD, PhD
Clinical Associate Professor, Division of geriatrics, Department of Internal Medicine,
Chonnam National University Bitgoeul Hospital, Gwang-ju, Republic of Korea

Sung Sun Kim, MD, PhD
Department of Pathology, Chonnam National University Medical School,
Gwangju, Republic of Korea

Ki-Hong Kim, MD
Department of Physical and Rehabilitation Medicine,
Chonnam National University Hospital & Medical School, Gwangju, Republic of Korea

Jonghwa Kim, MD, PhD
Department of Ophthalmology,
Chonnam National University Medical School, Gwangju, Republic of Korea

Jeonghwa Lee, PhD
Dean, College of Human Ecology, Chonnam National University
Professor, Department of Family Environment and Welfare,
Chonnam National University, Gwangju, Republic of Korea

Jeongjae Lee, PhD
Emeritus Professor, Department of Rural Systems Engineering, Seoul National University

Sungsu Lee, MD
Associate Professor, Department of Otolaryngology-Head and Neck Surgery,
Chonnam National University Medical School, Gwangju, Republic of Korea

Kichae Min, PhD
Professor, Department of Social Welfare,
Korea National University of Transportation, Chungcheong Buk-do, Republic of Korea

Kwangsung Park, MD, PhD
Director, Advanced Institute of Aging Science, Chonnam National University
Professor, Department of Urology, Chonnam National University Medical School,
Gwangju, Republic of Korea

Sang Chul Park, MD, PhD
Distinguished Professor, Chonnam National University, Gwangju, Republic of Korea
Chairman, International Centenarian Consortium (2005-2006)
President, International Association of Biomedical Gerontology (2003-2004)
Director, Seoul National University Institute on Aging (1996-2010)

Clara Yongjoo Park, PhD
Associate Professor, Division of Food and Nutrition, Chonnam National University,
Gwangju, Republic of Korea

Minho Shin, MD, PhD
Professor, Department of Preventive Medicine, Chonnam National University Medical School,
Gwangju, Republic of Korea

Kyung Chul Yoon, MD, PhD
Professor, Department of Ophthalmology, Chonnam National University Medical School,
Gwangju, Republic of Korea

Prologue

Why and How Does Korean Longevity Increase?

Sang Chul Park

South Korea became an aged society in 2017 and is expected to become a super-aged society by 2025. In addition, according to a paper by Mazid Ezzati *et al.* published in *Lancet* in 2017, it is predicted that the life expectancy of Korean women will exceed 90 years by 2030, and that they will have the greatest longevity in the world. Both in Korea and abroad, there is increasing interest in the future of super-aged societies and healthy longevity [Kontis *et al.*, 2017]. The two main fields of human aging research are longitudinal studies on aging and super-longevity research. While longitudinal studies on aging aim to understand the process and mechanisms of human aging by analyzing the phenomenon of aging in the flow of time and space in which humans live, super-longevity research aims to reveal the mechanisms of human life extension and health longevity by focusing mainly on super-aged people, including centenarians. Immortality and healthy longevity are the dreams of all human beings, and the people closest to these dreams are the super-agers that have managed to live over 100 years in relatively good health.

Historical Context

To understand the current state of longevity in Korea, it is essential to examine its historical context. South Korea has undergone significant political crises, including occupation by a foreign nation, World War II, and the Korean War. After these crises, the country experienced a great many socioeconomic and demographic changes. Through these changes, South Korea achieved rapid industrialization, urbanization, and improvements in the standard of living. These transformations have had a profound impact on the health and well-being of the population, and set the stage for increased longevity [Park SC, 2016].

Lifestyle Factors

Balanced Diet: Traditional Korean cuisine is known for its emphasis on vegetables, seafood, and fermented foods, combined with minimal use of red meat. This diet, which is rich in nutrients and low in unhealthy fats, has been crucial in promoting longevity. Additionally, the widespread consumption of kimchi, a fermented vegetable dish, has been linked to numerous health benefits due to its nutritional and probiotic properties.

Physical Activity: Koreans tend to engage in regular physical activity in their daily lives. Walking, hiking, and participating in traditional martial arts like Taekwondo are common activities that contribute to overall level of fitness in Korea. Regular exercise has been associated with a reduced risk of chronic diseases and increased life expectancy.

Strong Social Connections: Korean society strongly emphasizes community and familial ties. Social interactions and support networks have a positive impact on mental health and overall well-being, ultimately contributing to increased longevity.

Healthcare System

Universal National Healthcare: South Korea boasts a universal national healthcare system that provides all citizens with affordable access to medical services. This inclusive approach ensures that individuals can access preventive care, early diagnosis, and necessary treatments, leading to improved health outcomes and an increased life expectancy.

Advanced Medical Technology: The commitment to innovation and technological advancements has translated into significant progress in healthcare. South Korea is renowned for its cutting-edge medical technology and expertise, putting emphasis on areas such as telemedicine, robotic surgery, and stem cell research. These advancements have contributed to better healthcare outcomes and prolonged life expectancy.

Public Health Initiatives

Health Promotion: The Korean government has implemented various health promotion campaigns to raise awareness and to encourage healthy lifestyles among the population. These initiatives focus on smoking cessation, regular health check-ups, and disease prevention.

The government has had a positive impact on public health and longevity by targeting modifiable risk factors, such as tobacco use and unhealthy diets.

Elderly Care and Support: With an aging population, South Korea has implemented policies to support the well-being of older adults. These initiatives include healthcare programs, social welfare services, and infrastructure improvements to create an age-friendly environment. By addressing the needs of older adults, the government aims to enhance their quality of life and to extend their lifespan.

Cultural Factors

Work-Life Balance: The Korean conceptual agreement in terms of work-life balance emphasizes the importance of maintaining harmony between personal and professional lives. This cultural value encourages individuals to prioritize leisure, family time, and self-care, while reducing stress levels and contributing to improved overall health.

Respect for Elders: Korean society has a deep-rooted respect for elders, which extends to caregiving and support. Providing intergenerational care and transmitting wisdom and experiences across generations fosters a sense of purpose and belonging, positively impacting the mental and emotional well-being of Koreans.

Summary

The increase in Korean longevity can be attributed to a combination of lifestyle factors, a well-functioning healthcare system, public health initiatives, and cultural values. The emphases on a balanced diet, physical activity, strong social connections, and universal healthcare have been pivotal in improving health outcomes and extending life expectancy. Furthermore, the commitment of the Korean government to health promotion and support for older adults has created an environment that is conducive to longer and healthier lives. By understanding and learning from experience of Korea, it is hoped that other countries can adopt these strategies to enhance the longevity and well-being of their populations.

References

- Kontis V, Bennett JE, Mathers CD, Li G, Foreman K, Ezzati M. Future life expectancy in 35 industrialized countries: projections with a Bayesian model ensemble. Lancet 2017;389(10076):1323-1335.
- Park SC. Korean centenarian study: comprehensive approach for human longevity. In: Pachana NA. Encyclopedia of Geropsychology. Springer, Singapore: 2016. https://doi.org/10.1007/978-981-287-080-3_62-1.

Preface

Secrets and Changes in Korean Longevity

Kwangsung Park, Jae-Young Han, Jeonghwa Lee and Sang Chul Park

Welcome to the inaugural English edition of the Korean Centenarian Study, which follows in the footsteps of its predecessor, the *Korean centenarians: 20 years of change*, published in Korean in 2021. Spread across five enlightening sections, this book offers a comprehensive view of longevity in South Korea. This book consists of 5 parts and was contributed to by 19 authors.

Part Ⅰ, titled "Blue Zones and Korean Centenarians," delves into the global regions where people statistically enjoy the longest lifespans. Prof. Sang Chul Park, a trailblazer in Korean centenarian studies, provides an overview of the longevity belts in Korea. His findings in 2002 identified Gurye, Gokseong, Sunchang, and Damyang as longevity strongholds in South Korea, coining them the "GuGokSunDam Longevity Belt". Following this, Prof. Min Ho Shin elucidates the rapidly aging population of South Korea, emphasizing the dramatic rise in its elderly demographic. Closing this section, a deep dive into the prevalent diseases in older adults by Prof. Min-gu Kang illustrates the interplay between health and age.

Part Ⅱ examines the shifts in the family structures and elderly social welfare systems in South Korea. This section opens with an analysis by Prof. Jeonghwa Lee. She brings forth findings from centenarian studies, highlighting the societal shifts that have influenced the lives of centenarians in South Korea. Prof. Kichae Min brings to the forefront the shortcomings in the Korean welfare system and advocates taking a more positive view of increased longevity. Meanwhile, Prof. Minjeong An delves into the concept of gero-transcendence in Korean centenarians, a study aiming to influence policy and program development.

In Part Ⅲ, the health and lifestyle alterations of Korean centenarians are meticulously explored over seven chapters. The spotlight shines on the GuGokSunDam region, where Prof. Kwangsung Park and Min Jhon compare and contrast health data spanning nearly two decades. This section is further enriched by delving into the visual and auditory functions of centenarians, courtesy of insights from Prof. Kyung Chul Yoon, Hyong-Ho Cho, and their dedicated team. The following chapter analyzes lifestyle changes due to Korea's economic and technological ascent by Prof. Jae-Young Han. This is followed by an examination of dietary shifts over the past twenty years by Prof. Clara Yongjoo Park, the secrets of the centenarian immune system by Prof. Kyung A Cho, and the revelations of genetic characteristics by Prof. Sung Sun Kim.

Part Ⅳ offers readers an intimate glimpse into the lives of centenarians in the GuGokSunDam region. It contrasts insights gained from interviews conducted 20 years apart, portraying the daily realities of these longevity champions. A unique highlight is the remarkable journey of a semi-supercentenarian that faced and overcame numerous health challenges as she neared a century of life.

Finally, Part Ⅴ contemplates the future of a society blessed with longevity. This section resonates with lessons from the 2020 COVID-19 crisis, highlighting the vulnerabilities of older people. Prof. Sang Chul Park elucidates why older people were more affected and the survival of many centenarians, while reflecting upon the broader themes of aging. The closing chapter by Prof. Jung Jae Lee champions the potential of older people in the face of societal shifts, encouraging the younger generation to embrace an inclusive vision of the future, a vision where age is celebrated.

Settle in for a journey that unravels the many facets of longevity in Korea. Welcome to an exploration into a world where age is just a number, but the stories are timeless.

Contents

Lists of Contributors — 5

Prologue
Why and How Does Korean Longevity Increase?
Sang Chul Park — 7

Preface
Secrets and Changes in Korean Longevity
Kwangsung Park, Jae-Young Han, Jeonghwa Lee and Sang Chul Park — 13

Part I Blue Zones and Korean Centenarians

Chapter 01
History of Korean Centenarian Study
Background of Korean Longevity Belt Designation
Sang Chul Park — 23

Chapter 02
Trends in Aging of the Population in South Korea
Min Ho Shin — 29

Chapter 03
Trends of Disease Patterns in Older Adults
Min-gu Kang — 49

Part Ⅱ Changes in Family and Social Welfare System for Older People in Korea

Chapter 04
Changes in the Care and Family Systems of Korean Centenarians
Jeonghwa Lee —— 69

Chapter 05
Changes in the Social Welfare System for Older Adults in Korea
Kichae Min —— 85

Chapter 06
Gerotranscendence of Korean Centenarians
Minjeong An —— 101

Part Ⅲ Changes in Health Status and Lifestyle of Korean Centenarians

Chapter 07
Physical and Mental Health Status of Korean Centenarians
Kwangsung Park and Min Jhon —— 125

Chapter 08
Insights into the Visual Function of Korean Centenarians
Jonghwa Kim and Kyung Chul Yoon —— 137

Chapter 09
The Auditory Function of Korean Centenarians
Sungsu Lee and Hyong-Ho Cho —— 147

Chapter 10
Lifestyle Changes of Korean Centenarians
Ki-Hong Kim and Jae-Young Han —— 161

Chapter 11
Diets of Korean Centenarians
Clara Yongjoo Park —— 177

Chapter 12
The Immunity of Centenarians
the Secret to Maintaining a Healthy Llife and Surviving COVID-19
Kyung A Cho —— 199

Chapter 13
Genetics of Korean Centenarians
Sung Sun Kim —— 219

Part Ⅳ Case Studies of Korean Centenarians

Chapter 14
Special Cases of Centenarians in the GuGokSunDam Longevity Belt
Sang Chul Park, Kwangsung Park and Jeonghwa Lee —— 231

Chapter 15
A Special Case of the Medically Privileged Semisupercentenarian
Jeong Gwan Cho —— 247

Part Ⅴ Perspectives for Future Longlive Society

Chapter 16
Lessons from COVID-19 Crisis for New Normal in Future
Sang Chul Park —— 257

Chapter 17
Is there a Country for Old Men?
Jung Jae Lee —— 273

Epilogue

For a Better Future with a Longer Lifespan

Sang Chul Park, Jeonghwa Lee and Kwangsung Park — 279

PART I

BLUE ZONES AND KOREAN CENTENARIANS

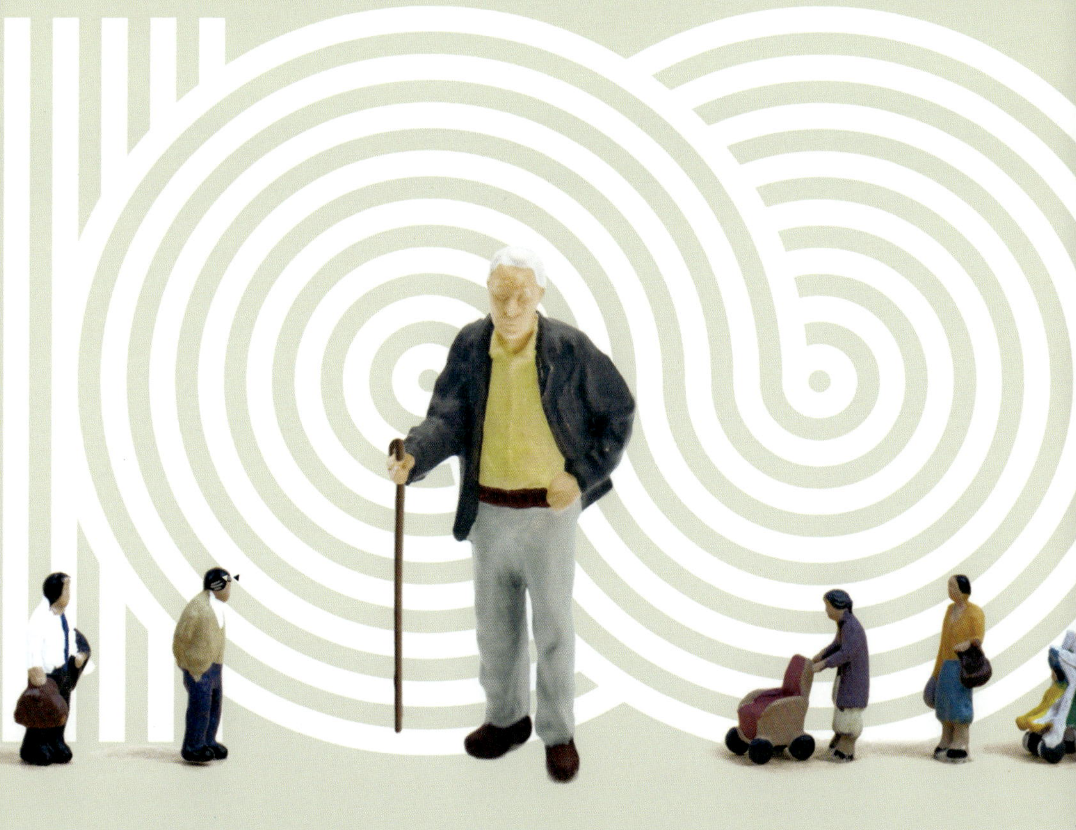

Chapter 01

History of Korean Centenarian Study

Background of Korean Longevity Belt Designation

Sang Chul Park

The study of centenarians and their longevity has always fascinated scientists and researchers worldwide. Understanding the factors that contribute to longevity can shed light on the secrets of longevity and help promote healthy aging in society. In South Korea, the study of centenarians has gained significant attention, leading to the designation of the Korean Longevity Belt. This chapter explores the history of the Korean centenarian study briefly and the background behind the designation of the Korean Longevity Belt.

Early Beginnings of Centenarian Study in Korea

The interest in studying centenarians in Korea can be traced back to the late 20th century when researchers began noticing a remarkable increase in the number of centenarians in the country. This rise in longevity was attributed to various factors, including healthcare improvements, nutrition, living conditions, *etc*. As the number of centenarians continued to grow, researchers recognized the need for a systematic study to understand the underlying causes.

Establishment of Centenarian Study Institutions

In the early 1990s, the Institute on Aging at Seoul National University was established to dedicate to the study of centenarians in Korea. The institution aimed to collect data, conduct comprehensive analyses, and identify factors associated with longevity. The research teams consisted of gerontologists, medical professionals, nutritionists, demographers, geographic economists, family study members, ecologists, and anthropologists, all working together to gain insights into the secrets of long life. The Korean Centenarians Study Group has been succeeded by the Korean Centenarian Study Group at the Advanced Institute of Aging Science at Chonnam National University.

Data Collection and Analysis

One of the key elements of the Korean centenarian study was the collection and analysis of comprehensive data. Research teams collaborated with local authorities, hospitals, community organizations, and Korea National Statistics Bureau to gather information on centenarians across the country. This included demographic data, medical records, lifestyle habits, and family history. The extensive data collection process provided a solid foundation for subsequent analyses.

Collaboration with International Research Institutions

Recognizing the importance of collaboration and knowledge exchange, Korean researchers actively sought partnerships with international institutions specializing in aging and longevity. Collaborations were established with renowned research centers in Japan, the United States, and European countries. These collaborations allowed for the comparison of findings and the adoption of best practices from around the world.

Identification of Key Factors

Through meticulous data analysis and extensive research, several key factors associated with longevity in Korea began to emerge. These factors included genetics, lifestyle choices, social connections, diet, and access to healthcare. Studies showed that certain regions in Korea had a higher concentration of centenarians, indicating the potential influence of environmental and cultural factors on longevity.

The Korean Longevity Belt Designation

Most people believe that the human lifespan is associated with the living environment. In fact, research on longevity regions has been conducted for a decade. In most studies on longevity regions, the focus has been on identifying the causes based on the natural environmental characteristics and dietary and lifestyle habits of these regions, mainly known as longevity villages. The common factors found in these regions were middle-high altitude areas with fluctuating terrain characterized by clear and not moist air. It is known that living in such areas demands a significant amount of physical activity, and they are regions where fresh fruits and vegetables can be consumed throughout the year[Park SC, 2002, 2012].

The Seoul National University Institute of Aging[Park SC *et al.*, 2008] selected longevity regions in South Korea based on specific criteria. Based on the number of centenarians and the proportion of the population over 85 years old among the elderly population, Gurye, Gokseong, Sunchang, and Damyang were designated as representative longevity regions in Korea and named the "GuGokSunDam Longevity Belt." These longevity belt regions have maintained their status as areas of longevity to this day, providing a platform for ongoing longitudinal studies on longevity[Park K *et al.*, 2021].

Implications and Applications

The designation of the Korean Longevity Belt brought about significant implications for public health, policy, and community development. It served as a platform for promoting healthy aging initiatives, both within and outside the designated areas. Local governments and community organizations in the Longevity Belt implemented programs to improve healthcare access, nutrition education, and social support for older adults. Furthermore, the findings from the Korean centenarian study influenced national policies on aging, contributing to the development of age-friendly cities and enhanced social welfare for older adults.

PART I

Summary

The history of the Korean centenarian study and the background behind the designation of the Korean Longevity Belt demonstrates the country's commitment to understanding and promoting healthy aging. Through collaboration, comprehensive data collection, and rigorous analysis, researchers have identified key factors associated with longevity and developed strategies for healthy aging initiatives. The Korean Longevity Belt serves as a beacon of inspiration, highlighting the potential for other regions to learn from its success in fostering a culture of longevity and promoting the well-being of older adults.

References

- Park K *et al.* Korean centenarians: 20 years of change. Koonja Publishing Inc., 2021.
- Park SC. Korean centenarian study. Seoul: Seoul National University Press, 2002.
- Park SC. Comprehensive approach for studying longevity in Korean centenarians. Asian J Gerontol Geriatr 2012;7:33-8.
- Park SC, Lee MS, Kwon IS, Kwak SC, Yeo EJ. Environment and gender influences on the nutritional and health status of Korean centenarians. Asian J Gerontology and Geriatrics. 2008;3(2):75-83.

Chapter 02

Trends in Aging of the Population in South Korea

Min Ho Shin

Population aging is the most important social change of the 21st century and will profoundly impact almost all areas of society, economy, politics, and culture. South Korea is experiencing one of the fastest aging populations in the world due to increasing life expectancy, rapidly declining fertility rates, and the entry of baby boomers into older adults. As a result of this rapid aging, the proportion of the population aged 65 and over has increased from 7.0% in 2000 to 10.9% in 2010 and 16.4% in 2020. South Korea needs to move faster to cope with the challenges of aging. In this chapter, we will look at the aging trend in South Korea and its main drivers: increasing life expectancy and declining fertility rates.

Trends and Causes of Population Aging

Trends in population aging

South Korea's population aging is progressing at the fastest rate globally. The United Nations (UN) defines 'elderly' as those aged 65 and over, categorizing societies based on the percentage of this age group: 'aging society' for 7% or more, 'aged society' for 14% or more, and 'post-aged society' for 20% or more. South Korea entered the aging society in 2000, the aged society in 2018, and is expected to become a post-aged society by 2025. The speed of aging in Korea is unprecedentedly rapid. It took Korea only 18 years to move from 7% to 14% of the elderly population, while it took France 115 years, the US 73 years, Germany 40 years, and even Japan, known for its rapid aging, 24 years. Over the last decade, South Korea's elderly population (aged 65 and over) has been growing at an annual average of 4.4%, which is significantly higher than the OECD average of 2.6%, making it the fastest among OECD countries. The proportion of older people in South Korea

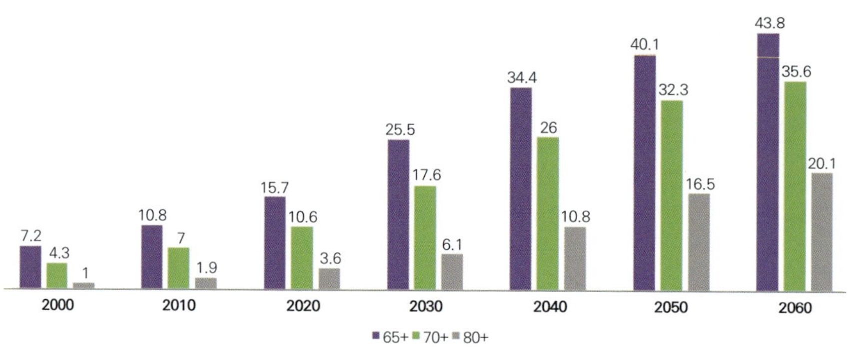

Figure 2-1. Trends and projections of the elderly population in Korea, 2000–2060

fastest worldwide, the proportion of South Korea's elderly population is expected to increase rapidly from 15.7% in 2020 to 34.4% in 2040 and 43.8% in 2060. The percentage of people aged 80 and over was 1% in 2000 and 3.6% in 2020, and it is expected to increase rapidly to 10.8% in 2040 and 20.1% in 2060. As a result, the number of older people is expected to rise from 8.12 million in 2020 to 17.24 million in 2040 and 18.68 million in 2060(Figure 2-1).

According to the 2022 World Population Prospects [United Nations, 2022], the proportion of the elderly population in South Korea was 13.1% in 2015, making it an aging society alongside countries like Mexico, Turkey, and Chile. However, during the same year, countries like Japan, Italy, Greece, and Germany had already entered the post-aged society stage. As the rate of aging in Korea is currently the

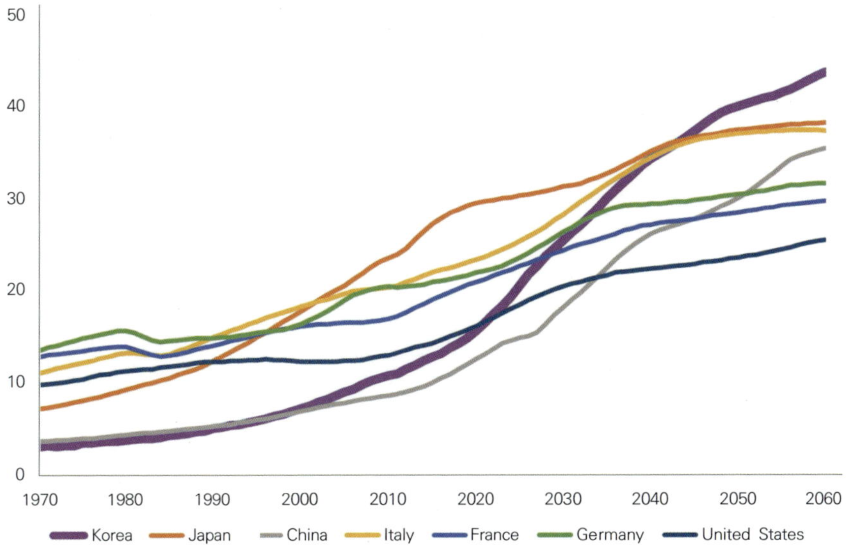

Figure 2-2. Estimated and projected population ratio aged 65 and over in major countries, 1970-2060

surpassed that of the United States in 2022. It is expected to sur pass that of France by 2028, Germany by 2035, Italy by 2042, and Japan by 2044(Figure 2-2).

The population pyramid of Korea has been evolving over the years. In 1960 and 1980, it took the shape of a triangle with a high population density of children and teenagers. By 2000, the population pyramid resembled a bell shape with a higher population density in the 30-40 age group. By 2020, it took the shape of a vase with a higher population density in the 50-60 age group. The projection for 2040 shows an inverted triangle shape due to a higher population density of older people, and by 2060, the proportion of the population over 80 years old is expected to be so high that the pyramid will display a pronounced inverted triangle shape(Figure 2-3) [Statistics Korea, 2022].

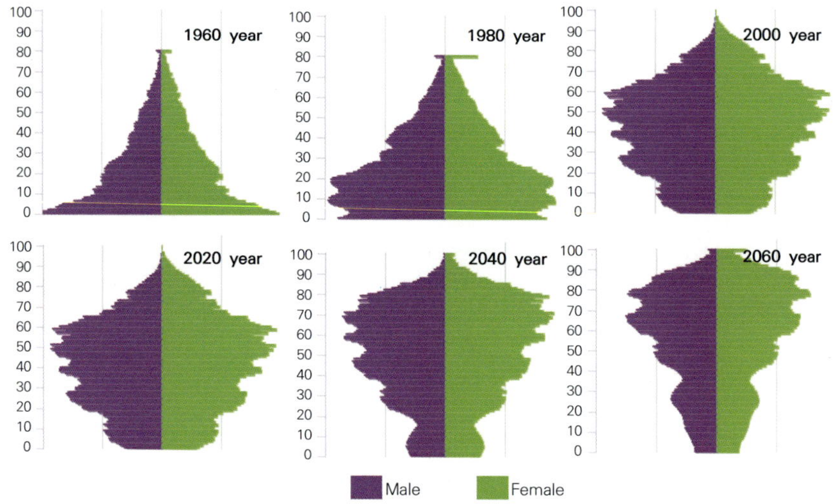

Figure 2-3. Population pyramids of South Korea by period

Increase in life expectancy

- Comparison of domestic and international trends

The increase in life expectancy is one of the main factors accelerating population aging. Over the past century, life expectancy has significantly improved worldwide, with the global average life expectancy rising from 45.5 years in 1950 to 72.6 years in 2020. The life expectancy of Koreans was 62.3 years in 1970, lower than the OECD member states' average life expectancy of 70 years, but it surpassed the OECD average after 2005. In 2020, the life expectancy of Korean men was 80.3 years, 2.5 years higher than the OECD average of 77.9 years. Korean women's life expectancy was 86.3 years, 3.1 years higher than the OECD average of 83.2 years. Korea has the second-highest life expectancy among the 37 OECD member states, following Japan [OECD, 2023b]. According to UN population projections, the life expectancy for individuals aged 65 is expected to increase from 17 years in 2015-2020 to 19 years in 2045-2050(Figure 2-4).

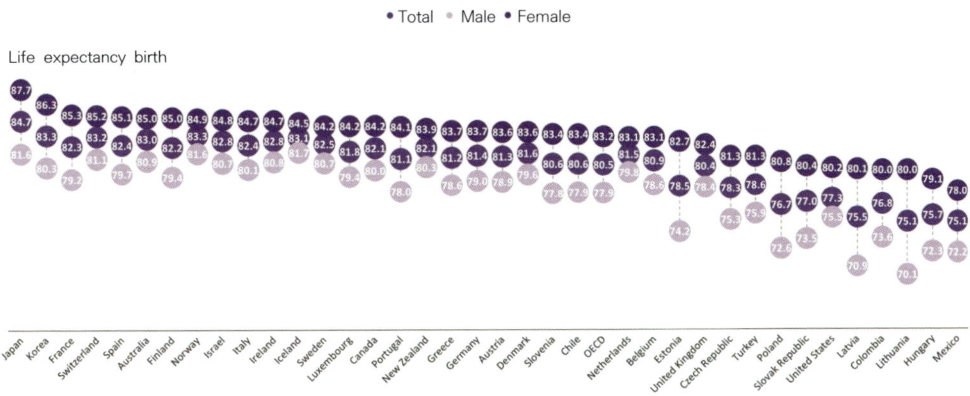

Figure 2-4. Life expectancy in OECD member countries, 2020 or the latest available year

The life expectancy in Korea has been continuously increasing for the past 50 years. From 1970, it increased at an annual average of 0.47 years for 40 years, and then by 0.32 years over the next 20 years. The life expectancy of Koreans is expected to continue to rise. In 2019, the life expectancy of Koreans was 83.3 years, but by around 2060, it is predicted to increase to 89.4 years. The gender gap in life expectancy peaked at 8.6 years in 1985, but decreased to 6.0 years in 2019, and is projected to further shrink to 3.4 years by 2060(Figure 2-5) [Statistics Korea, 2022].

The gender gap in life expectancy is a phenomenon that appears in almost every country. According to the World Population Prospects 2019, the life expectancy of women was 4.6 years higher than that of men. The difference in life expectancy between genders varied by region, with Latin America and the Caribbean showing a large gap of 6.5 years, Europe and North America 6.1 years, Southeast Asia 5.3 years, while Central Asia had a smaller gap of 2.7 years,

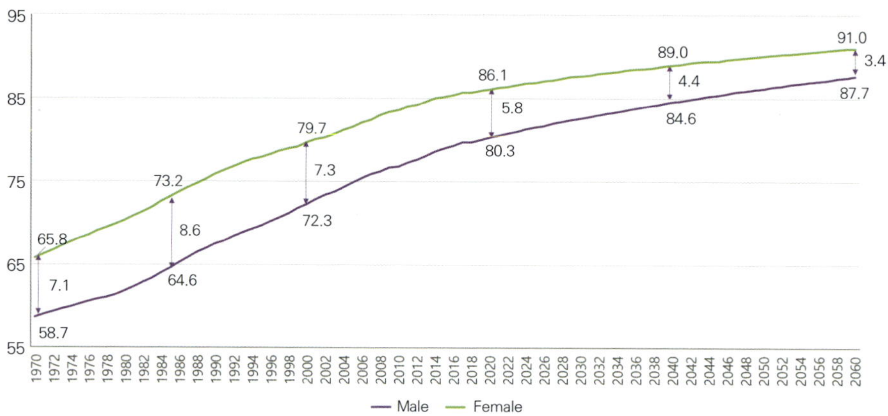

Figure 2-5. Life expectancy and the gender difference in life expectancy in South Korea

Oceania 3.0 years, and SubSaharan Africa 3.5 years. When looking at the gap by country, the gap was even greater, with Russia having the largest difference of 10 years and Bhutan the smallest at 0.5 years. The gender gap in life expectancy in Korea was 6.0 years, higher than the OECD average of 5.3 years and the global average of 4.6 years.

The factors explaining the gender difference in life expectancy include biological factors, health behavior factors, and environmental factors, and it has not been revealed how much each factor contributes relatively. The fact that the gender difference in life expectancy varies greatly by country and changes over time suggests that biological differences may not be significant. It is expected that the gender gap in life expectancy in Korea will decrease due to changes in health behaviors and environmental factors that influence the gender difference in life expectancy. The gender gap in life expectancy in Korea is currently 6.0 years and is expected to decrease to 3.4 years by 2060.

While women generally live longer than men, most of this increased life expectancy is spent in poor health. Life table data from Statistics Korea offers some insights. For babies born in 2018, the chronic disease-free life expectancy was 64.4 years, and life expectancy in perceived good health was 69.0 years. There was a gender difference in overall life expectancy of 6 years. However, the chronic disease-free life expectancy showed a smaller difference: 64.0 years for men and 64.9 years for women, a difference of just 0.9 years. Furthermore, the difference in life expectancy in perceived good health was even smaller: 69.1 years for men compared to 69.0 years for women, a difference of a mere 0.1 years.

Decline in birthrate

The number of newborns in South Korea exceeded 1 million until the early 1970s, but it has continuously decreased since then, reaching the level of 600,000 to 700,000 in the 1980s and 1990s. Furthermore, it shrank to 400,000 after 2001 and remained at this level until 2015, but from 2016 onwards, it decreased by more than 10% each year, with the number of births in 2022 falling to 249,000. The birthrate is typically measured by the total fertility rate, which is the ratio of the number of births to the average number of women of childbearing age (15-49 years old) per year. The level of the total fertility rate that can maintain the current population is called the population replacement rate, which is about

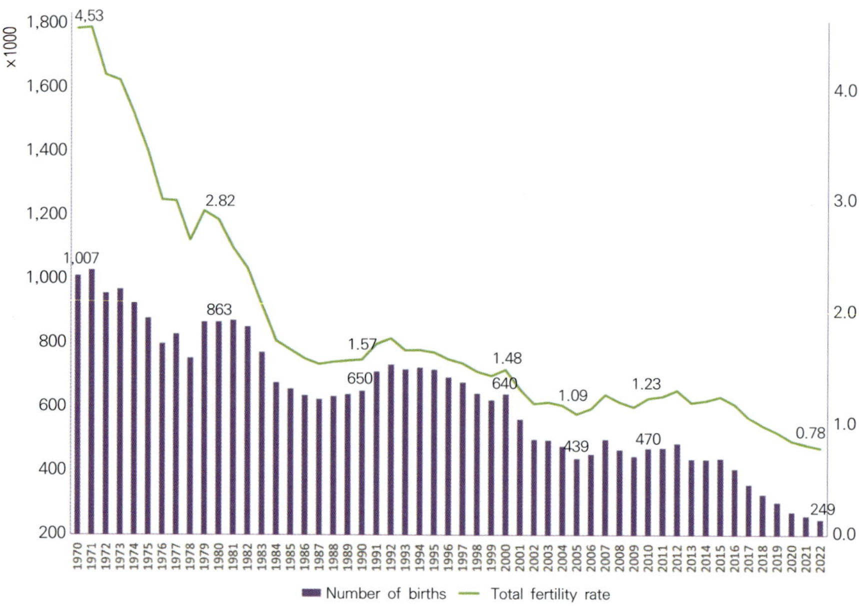

Figure 2-6. Trends in the number of births and total fertility rate in South Korea, 1970-2022

2.1 according to OECD and UN standards. The total fertility rate was at a level of 6.0 in 1960, but it dramatically decreased due to the introduction of the family planning project, a birth control policy in the 1960s. Although it remained high at 4.5 in the 1970s, it dropped to the population replacement level of 2.1 in 1983, and has continued to decline ever since, reaching 1.08 in 2005. It drastically fell from 2016 onwards, decreasing to 0.78 in 2022(Figure 2-6) [Statistics Korea, 2023b].

The total fertility rate in South Korea is the lowest in the world and the lowest among the OECD member countries. Compared to other OECD member countries, South Korea's total fertility rate was the fourth highest in 1960, but it rapidly decreased and became lower than the OECD average from 1983, and in 2004, it had the lowest rank among the OECD member countries. As of 2021, the average total fertility rate for the 37 OECD member countries was 1.60. South Korea was the only country with a figure below 1, exhibiting a rate of 0.81. Israel had the highest fertility rate among OECD member countries at 3.00, followed by the Czech Republic and Mexico at 1.83 and 1.82, respectively. Other countries with low fertility rates included Spain with 1.19, and Italy with 1.25. The fertility rates for major developed countries were 1.66 for the United States, 1.53 for the United Kingdom, 1.58 for Germany, and 1.30 for Japan(Figures 2-7 and 2-8).

The total fertility rates in most OECD member countries, excluding Israel and Mexico, show a trend of decreasing to levels below the population replacement rate, then rebounding. The fertility rate in France fell to 1.60 in 1993 but rebounded to 2.02 by 2010. In Sweden, the rate dropped to 1.50 in 1999 but bounced back to 1.98 by 2010. Countries recovering at a relatively slower pace include Germany and Japan. Germany's fertility rate fell to 1.24 in

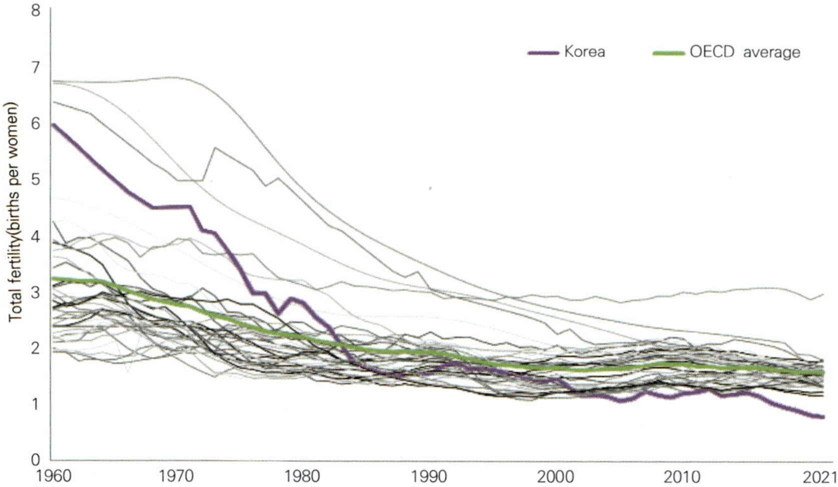

Figure 2-7. Trends in the total fertility rate of OECD member countries, 1960-2021

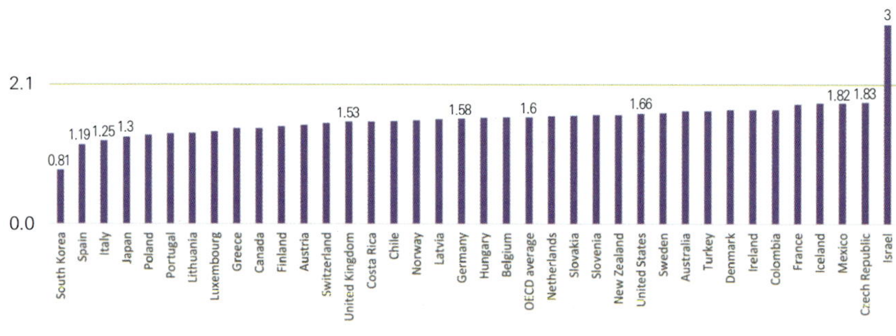

Figure 2-8. Comparison of the total fertility rates of OECD member countries, 2021

1994 but rebounded to 1.59 by 2016. In Japan, the rate fell to 1.24 in 2005 but rose to 1.46 by 2015(Figure 2-9) [OECD, 2023a].

In South Korea, the decrease in the number of marriages and the rise in the age of first marriage are important factors contributing to low birth rates. The number of marriages held steady at

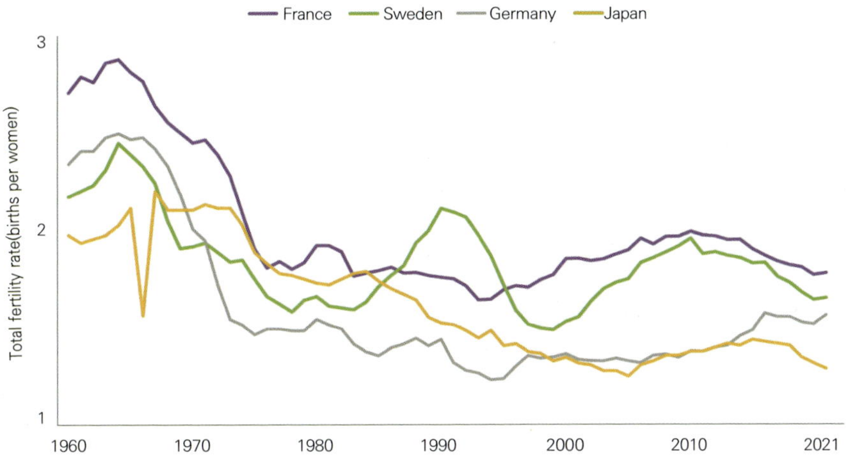

Figure 2-9. OECD member countries showing a rebound in the downward trend of total fertility rates

around 400,000 from 1980 to 1996, reaching its peak at 434,911 in 1996. From the late 1990s, this number began to decline, rapidly decreasing from 2016 onwards. By 2020, the number of marriages had dropped to 213,502, half of the figure from 1996. The crude marriage rate, which represents the number of marriages per 1,000 people, also declined over the same period. It was highest in 1980 at 10.6 but steadily decreased to 3.7 by 2022 [Statistics Korea, 2023a]. Notably, in 2020-2022, the number dropped significantly compared to the previous year due to the impact of the COVID-19 pandemic. This decrease is attributed to an increase in people postponing or canceling their weddings due to restrictions on gatherings amid intensified social distancing measures(Figure 2-10).

An increase in the age at first marriage can delay the birth of a first child and shorten the reproductive period, leading to decreased fertility rates. The age of first marriage for women is rising worldwide.

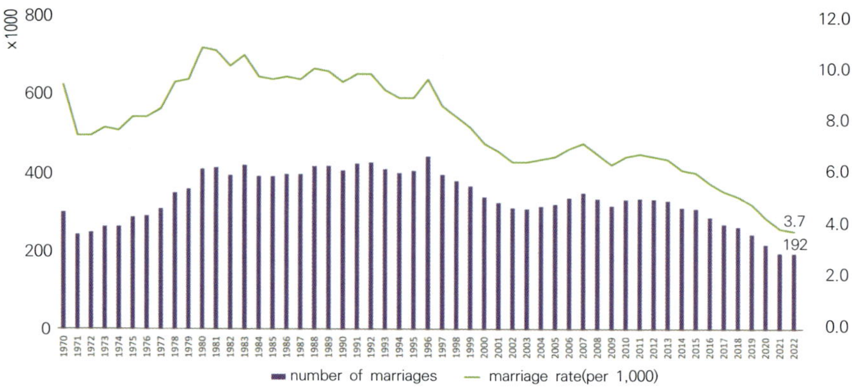

Figure 2-10. Trends in the number of marriages and crude marriage rate in South Korea, 1970-2022

In OECD countries, the average age at first marriage in the early 1990s was 25 for women and 27 for men, which rose to 30 for women and 32 for men by 2016. South Korea was below the OECD average in the 1990s, but increased to a level close to the OECD average in the 2010s and has continued to rise since then. From 1970 to 1990, the age at first marriage for men increased by 0.7 years, from 27.1 to 27.8, while the age at first marriage for women increased by 1.5 years, from 23.3 to 24.8. Since 1995, the increase has been larger for men, 4.8 years for men and 5.5 years for women, but the increase is still 0.7 years larger for women. The age at first marriage was 27.8 years for men and 24.8 years for women in 1990, and has steadily increased since then, reaching 29.3 years for men and 26.5 years for women in 2000, 31.8 years for men and 28.9 years for women in 2010, and 33.7 years for men and 31.3 years for women in 2022(Figure 2-11) [Statistics Korea, 2023a].

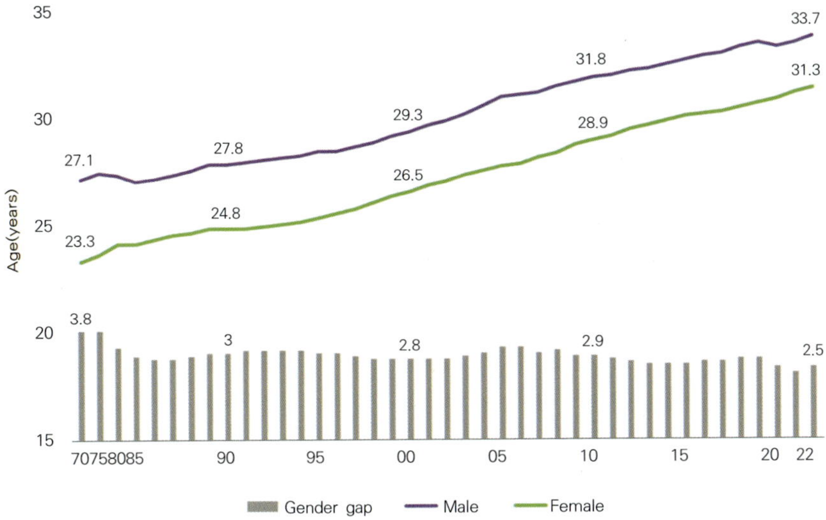

Figure 2-11. Trends in age at first marriage in South Korea, 1970-2022

Population decline

Despite a recent decrease in birth rates, the absolute size of South Korea's population has continued to increase due to the greater impact of rising life expectancy. However, since 2020, a natural decrease in population, where the number of deaths exceeds the number of births, has begun due to a drastic reduction in the number of newborns based on domestic residents (Figure 2-12) [Statistics Korea, 2023b]. According to Statistics Korea's future population estimate, the population of South Korea is expected to increase from 51.78 million in 2020 to 51.94 million in 2028, then decrease to 50.86 million in 2040 and 42.83 million in 2067. Among these, the domestic population is projected to decrease from 50.05 million in 2020 to 48.58 million in 2040. International migration plays an important role in population change, and foreigners, who accounted for 3.3% of the total population at 1.73 million in 2020, are projected

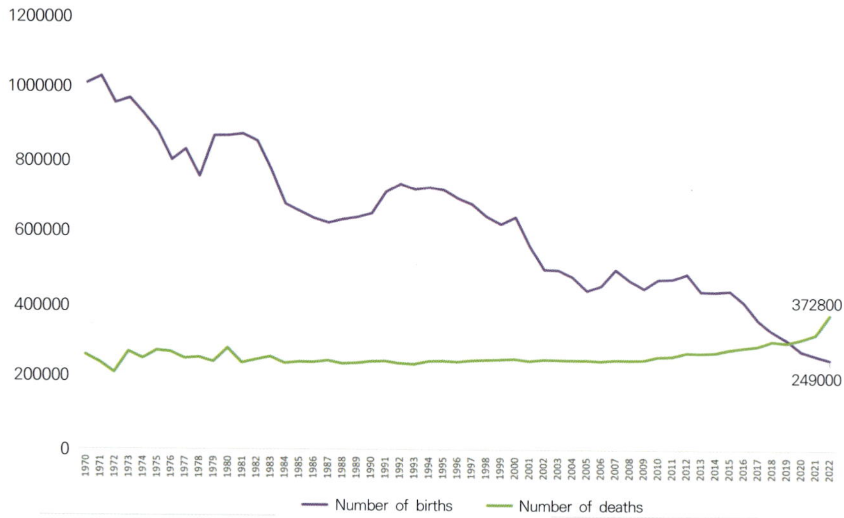

Figure 2-12. Trends in the number of births and deaths in South Korea, 1970-2022

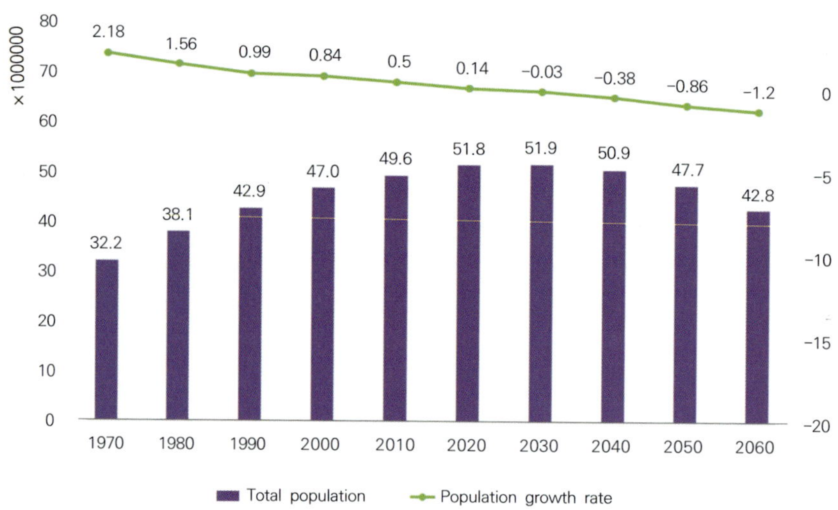

Figure 2-13. Trends in population size and population growth rate in South Korea, 1970-2060

to continuously increase to 2.28 million, accounting for 4.5% of the total in 2040(Figure 2-13) [Statistics Korea, 2022].

However, these population projections could potentially be somewhat optimistic. The 2019 population projection estimated total fertility rates for 2019, 2020, and 2021 at 0.94, 0.90, and 0.86, respectively, but the actual total fertility rates for these years were 0.92, 0.84, and 0.81, respectively. This suggests that the trend of population decline among the domestic population could be proceeding more rapidly than expected.

Impacts of Aging Population and Countermeasures

The aging population in South Korea is increasing at the fastest rate in the world, and the elderly population is expected to increase both relatively and absolutely in the future. The proportion of the elderly population in South Korea is projected to increase from 15.7% in 2020 to 33.9% in 2040, and 43.9% in 2060 [Statistics Korea, 2022]. The median age is also expected to rise from 43.7 years in 2020 to 54.4 years in 2040 and 61.3 years in 2060. The old-age dependency ratio is expected to increase from 21.7 per 100 people in 2020 to 60.1 in 2040, and 91.4 in 2060, a 4.2-fold increase over 20 years. The elderly population will increase from 8.12 million in 2020 to 17.22 million in 2040, and 18.81 million by 2060. As a result of rapid aging and an absolute increase in the elderly population, economic growth is expected to slow down, and the fiscal burden is anticipated to increase. A decrease in the productive population will likely lead to a decrease in government revenue, while public expenditures such as social welfare services, pensions, and medical costs are projected to rise. Especially, with rapid aging, healthcare costs are expected to surge dramatically due to an increase in chronic disease patients. Korea's healthcare expenditure as a percentage of GDP rose from 6.5% in 2014 to 8% in 2019, an increase of 1.5%, but the OECD average only increased by 0.1% from 8.7% to 8.8% during the same period. The proportion of elderly medical expenses in total healthcare costs increased by 9.3% from 32.3% in 2010 to 41.6% in 2019, accounting for 41% of total healthcare expenses of KRW 86.5 trillion in 2019. Elderly medical expenses have been increasing by more than 10% annually since 2014, and increased by 13.2% in 2019. If the increase in medical expenses due to aging is not curbed, it will be impossible to maintain a sustainable medical system. To curb the rise in medical expenses for the elderly, the healthcare system should transition from being treatment-centered to focusing on disease prevention and health promotion. Additionally, the medical payment system needs to be reformed to ensure sustainable health insurance.

In Korea, the issue of a low birthrate is considered the most important cause of rapid aging. The 4th Basic Plan for Low Fertility and Aging Society in 2020 identifies socio-economic factors, cultural values, and demographic factors as causes of low fertility in Korea [Low Birth Rate and Aged Society Committee, 2020]. Socio-economic factors include an unstable job market, intensified competition in education, high housing prices, a genderbiased labor market, and a lack of care infrastructure. Cultural value factors include the persistence of traditional family norms, and changes in the perception of marriage and children among young people. Demographic factors include the decrease in the population of women of childbearing age, the continued decline in marriage rates and the increase in first marriage age, and the decrease in the average number of births and increase in the percentage of childless households among married couples. The Korean government's low birthrate policy, implemented since the mid-1990s, failed to prevent the birth rate decline as it focused on encouraging birth rather than policies accompanied by social structural changes. It's time to implement bold policies to solve the structural problems of Korean society that affect birth rates, such as high housing and education costs, employment instability, generational income gap, and inadequate childcare environments. In 2006, a European demographer, Wolfgang Lutz, proposed the "low fertility trap" hypothesis to explain the ultra-low fertility phenomenon in Korea and Japan. He pointed out that once a country falls into the trap of low fertility, it's difficult to escape unless drastic measures are taken [Lutz W. *et al.*, 2006]. Countries like France and Sweden, which have seen a rebound in birth rates, successfully boosted birth rates by actively implementing family policies based on gender equality and inclusiveness at the point where the total fertility rate fell to its lowest level. In Korea, there's also a need for proactive promotion of gender-equal family policies that can alleviate young people's avoidance of marriage and childbirth. During the recent COVID-19 pandemic, the number of marriages sharply decreased due to social distancing policies, exacerbating the problem of low birthrate. The pandemic has also rapidly changed the values of young people towards marriage and childbirth, and the negative impact on fertility rates is likely to appear long-term. In the post-COVID era, more aggressive measures against low fertility are needed for sustainable growth.

To address the rapid aging problem, it is crucial to construct a society friendly to active and healthy aging. Healthy aging refers to the process of ensuring opportunities to appropriately maintain physical, social, and mental health, despite advancing age, enabling individuals to lead independent and fulfilling lives without discrimination based on age or gender, and to participate in social activities actively. Maintaining healthy lifestyle habits or improving unfavorable ones in old age is critical in preventing diseases and disabilities. Especially in old age, physical activity is one of the most important determinants of health, and maintaining an active state is key to sustaining health, mobility, and independence. However, according to the Korea National Health and Nutrition Examination Survey, physical activity in older people is continuously decreasing. The practice rate of walking has significantly decreased yearly, from 54.6% in 2005 to 33.5% in 2012, although it has slightly increased since then to 39.6% in 2019. There is a need to establish a national infrastructure to increase physical activity among older people. In order to create an age-friendly environment, housing, transportation, and living environments that consider the needs of older people should be provided. Customized housing based on the degree of aging and easily accessible transportation are the most essential elements that enable older people to maintain independent lives and facilitate interactions with other members of society, thus allowing them to function as members of society.

Summary

Population aging is the most important social change of the 21st century and will profoundly impact almost all areas of society, economy, politics, and culture. The country is expected to enter a post-aged society by 2025, with the elderly population ratio projected to increase to 34.4% by 2040. Key factors behind this trend include a rise in life expectancy and a decline in birth rates. Notably, South Korea ranks second in life expectancy among OECD member countries but has one of the world's lowest fertility rates. This demographic shift raises concerns about economic slowdown and increasing financial burdens. There's an emerging need to reform the healthcare system towards disease prevention and to establish a sustainable health insurance system. To address the challenges of rapid aging, it is imperative for South Korea to cultivate a society that encourages active and healthy aging, and to create age-friendly environments.

References

- Low Birth Rate and Aged Society Committee (2020), The 4th Basic Plan for Low Birth Rate and Aged Society: 2021～2025.
- Lutz, Wolfgang, Vegard Skirbekk, and Maria Rita Testa. 2006. The low-fertility trap hypothesis: Forces that may lead to further postponement and fewer births in Europe. Vienna yearbook of population research:167-192.
- OECD (2023a), Fertility rates (indicator).
doi: 10.1787/8272fb01-en (Accessed on 26 June 2023)
- OECD (2023b), Life expectancy at birth (indicator).
doi: 10.1787/27e0fc9d-en (Accessed on 26 June 2023)
- Statistics Korea (2022). Population Projections for Korea (2020～2070)
- Statistics Korea (2023a). Marriage and Divorce Statistics in 2022.
- Statistics Korea (2023b). Preliminary Results of Birth and Death Statistics in 2022.
- United Nations, Department of Economic and Social Affairs, Population Division (2022). World Population Prospects 2022, Online Edition.

Chapter 03

Trends of Disease Patterns in Older Adults

Min-gu Kang

Introduction

The most straightforward method of evaluating one's health status is by assessing the presence of disease. However, there are numerous types of diseases, and their severity can vary significantly. According to the National Survey of Living Conditions and Welfare Needs of Older Koreans 2017 conducted by the Ministry of Health and Welfare in Korea, about 90% of older individuals suffer from one or more chronic diseases, with more than half of them having three or more chronic illnesses [The Korean Society of Geriatrics, 2018]. Consequently, when examining disease trends among the older population, it is essential to concentrate on significant diseases that considerably impact health.

Here, we would like to define the significant diseases as the following two types: Firstly, diseases that are major causes of death, as the ultimate loss of health due to disease is death. Secondly, diseases that result in functional decline and reduce the period of healthy living. The WHO constitution defines health as 'a state of complete physical, mental, and social well-being and not merely the absence of disease or infirmity.' However, expecting older individuals to achieve such a state in reality is challenging. Therefore, it is necessary to focus on the functional status when considering the meaning of health. For instance, an older person with hypertension, hyperlipidemia, and diabetes who regularly visits the hospital and takes medication but can still manage daily activities such as shopping, using transportation, and managing finances may appear to be in good health. However, another older person who has suffered a stroke and is paralyzed on one side of the body, has difficulty walking, and requires assistance with dressing and bathing is clearly facing serious health challenges that require constant care. In other words, the presence or absence of functional limitations is crucial in assessing health status, as these limitations can greatly diminish quality of life. Therefore, identifying diseases that affect functional status is as important as identifying those that cause death. Based on the two criteria described above, we would like to describe the trend of disease patterns in older adults.

Changes in the Major Causes of Death from Diseases Among the Older Adults

In this chapter, we aim to examine the changes in diseases that are the primary cause of death in the older population from 2000 to 2019. Our analysis will start by looking at the changes in diseases that are the leading causes of death globally, and then we will shift our focus to diseases that are prevalent in Korea. Identifying such diseases is critical to reducing mortality rates among the older population. Consequently, efforts are needed to develop effective prevention strategies to address these diseases.

PART I

Changes in the major causes of death from diseases worldwide

According to data from the World Health Organization (WHO), (Table 3-1), ischemic heart disease has been the leading cause of death worldwide for the past 20 years [Park K *et al.*, 2021]. This disease occurs when there is a disruption in the adequate blood supply to the heart due to disorders in the coronary artery blood flow. The two main types of ischemic heart disease are angina pectoris and myocardial infarction. Ischemic heart disease has been responsible for more than 20% of all deaths worldwide in people over the age of 70 during the last two decades.

The prominent change in causes of death is the emergence of dementia, including Alzheimer's disease, as a major cause of death [Park K *et al.*, 2021]. In 2000, dementia, including Alzheimer's disease, accounted for around 2.70% of the major causes of death, but in 2019, it accounted for 5.65% of the major causes of death. The proportion of deaths caused by dementia has more than doubled, and the actual number of deaths has increased by about three times. As a result, dementia, including Alzheimer's disease, has risen to the fifth leading cause of death among older adults in 2019.

Alzheimer's disease is known as the most common cause of dementia, a degenerative brain disorder. The disease develops slowly and progressively. In the early stages of the disease, patients often show memory impairment, and as the disease progresses, they exhibit overall cognitive dysfunction, ultimately losing all their daily life functions. Alzheimer's disease usually occurs after age 65, and advanced age is a major risk factor for its development. Considering the global trend of increasing life expectancy, the importance of Alzheimer's disease is expected to become more prominent in the future.

Malignant neoplasm is a disease that is becoming increasingly prevalent as one of the leading causes of death, ranking second in 2019 [Park K *et al.*, 2021]. The incidence of malignant neoplasm tends to increase with age, although this varies depending on the type of malignant neoplasm. The causes of malignant neoplasm have been linked to various factors such as prolonged exposure to carcinogens, decreased ability to repair DNA damage, activation of oncogenes, reduced function of tumor suppressor genes, and weakened immune function. Similar to Alzheimer's disease, malignant neoplasm is expected to become increasingly important as the human lifespan continues to increase.

Hypertensive heart disease, diabetes mellitus, and chronic kidney disease are among the major causes of death in older adults and are gradually increasing over time [Park K *et al.*, 2021]. It is important to give these diseases special attention as they are directly linked to the management of chronic diseases. Hypertensive heart disease occurs due to long-term high blood pressure, leading to heart structure changes. This risk can be reduced by properly managing blood pressure through lifestyle changes and medication. Diabetes mellitus is a metabolic disease characterized by a rise in blood sugar levels due to inadequate insulin secretion or insulin resistance. It also requires lifestyle changes and medication to manage. Failure to control blood sugar levels can lead to severe acute complications that can be life-threatening and require urgent treatment. In addition, diabetes mellitus can also lead to chronic complications such as retinopathy, nephropathy, neuropathy, coronary artery disease, and cerebrovascular disease. Chronic kidney disease is a medical condition characterized by a continuous decline in kidney function. It can be diagnosed after confirming decreased renal function over a period of three months or more. This condition is closely linked to chronic diseases like diabetes mellitus and hypertension, which are the most common causes of chronic kidney disease. Proper management and treatment of these underlying conditions, such as controlling hypertension, managing diabetes mellitus, and addressing hyperlipidemia, is crucial in preventing the onset and progression of chronic kidney disease.

Stroke is a significant cause of death, accounting for 14.80% of all causes of death among older adults in 2019. However, the rate of stroke-related deaths has gradually decreased over time, from 17.67% in 2000 [Park K *et al.*, 2021]. There are two types of strokes: cerebral infarction caused by blockage of cerebral blood vessels and cerebral hemorrhage caused by rupture of cerebral blood vessels. Of the two types, the reduction in cerebral hemorrhage is more pronounced, particularly in countries with high-income levels. Diarrheal disease is also a leading cause of death, although its importance as a cause of death is declining. The excretion of soft and watery stools characterizes diarrhea. Diarrheal disease, which is the cause of death, is mainly caused by infection with viruses, bacteria, or parasites. To prevent this disease, it is crucial to consume safe water, such as by boiling or treating it, and practice proper hygiene, such as washing hands before and after preparing and consuming food.

One of the major causes of death among older adults is chronic obstructive pulmonary disease (COPD) [Park K *et al.*, 2021]. COPD is a respiratory disease characterized by persistent airflow limitation, dyspnea, cough, and sputum due to abnormalities in the airways and alveoli. Smoking is the leading cause of COPD, but continuous exposure to harmful substances such as gas, smoke, and chemicals at work can also lead to COPD. Quitting smoking is the most effective way to prevent COPD and slow down the progression of the disease. However, apart from smoking cessation, several efforts such as drug treatment, influenza vaccination, and respiratory rehabilitation are necessary to alleviate symptoms and prevent acute deterioration. Lower respiratory tract infections are another major cause of death among older adults. Pneumonia is caused by microorganisms, including bacteria, viruses, and fungi, and it is the

Table 3-1. **Changes in the top 10 causes of death from diseases among older adults worldwide** (Global Health Estimate 2019: Deaths by Cause, Age, Sex, by Country and Region, 2000-2019. Geneva, World Health Organization; 2020.) Abbreviation: COPD, chronic obstructive pulmonary disease.

Ranking	2000	2010	2015	2019	Note
1	Ischemic heart disease	Ischemic heart disease	Ischemic heart disease	Ischemic heart disease	
2	Stroke	Stroke	Malignant neoplasm	Malignant neoplasm	
3	Malignant neoplasm	Malignant neoplasm	Stroke	Stroke	
4	COPD	COPD	COPD	COPD	
5	Lower respiratory tract infection	Lower respiratory tract infection	Alzheimer's disease, dementia	Alzheimer's disease, dementia	
6	Diarrheal disease	Alzheimer's disease, dementia	Lower respiratory tract infection	Lower respiratory tract infection	
7	Alzheimer's disease, dementia	Diarrheal disease	Hypertensive heart disease	Hypertensive heart disease	
8	Hypertensive heart disease	Hypertensive heart disease	Diabetes mellitus	Diabetes mellitus	
9	Diabetes mellitus	Diabetes mellitus	Chronic kidney disease	Chronic kidney disease	
10	Chronic kidney disease	Chronic kidney disease	Diarrheal disease	Diarrheal disease	

most frequent type of lower respiratory tract infection. Due to the increased risk for severe pneumonia in older adults, its importance is becoming more apparent in countries with rapidly aging populations.

Changes in the major causes of death from diseases in the domestic population

The World Bank categorizes countries based on their Gross National Income (GNI) per capita into four groups: low-income countries, lower-middle-income countries, upper-middle-income countries, and high-income countries. In 2000, Korea had a per capita GNI of $10,740, which was on the border between upper-middle-income and high-income countries. However, in 2019, Korea had a per capita GNI of over $30,000 and became a central high-income

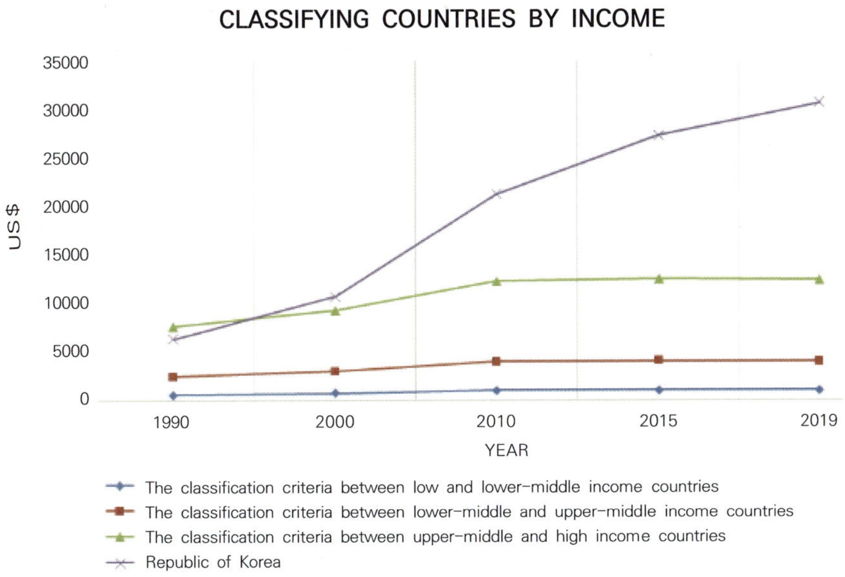

Figure 3-1. Changes in the Republic of Korea's status in the country classification by gross national income per capita (Classifying countries by income, The World Bank; 2019.)

country.(Figure 3-1) This reflects the significant economic growth and development that Korea has experienced over the past two decades. Interestingly, the leading cause of death among older adults in Korea in 2000 was stroke, which was also the number 1 cause of death in the upper-middle-income group. However, in 2019, the number 1 cause of death among older adults in Korea was malignant neoplasm, which is also the number 1 cause of death in the high-income group. This suggests that as a country becomes more developed and affluent, the leading causes of death may shift from diseases associated with poverty and lack of access to healthcare to diseases related to lifestyle and aging.

The prevalence of stroke as a cause of death among older adults has significantly decreased from 23.71% to 9.71%.(Figure 3-2) This decrease in mortality rates can be attributed to improved management of chronic diseases and the development of emergency care systems. For example, there has been a marked increase in blood pressure control rates among hypertensive patients aged 70 years or older. According to the Korea National Health and Nutrition Examination Survey conducted in 2001, the blood pressure control rate among hypertensive patients aged 70 years or older was 11.6% for men and 17.9% for women. However, in the Korea National Health and Nutrition Examination Survey conducted in 2019, the rate of blood pressure control in the same age group was 62.9% for men and 51.1% for women [Korean Society of Hypertension, 2020]. Moreover, Korea designated 18 medical institutions as regional emergency medical centers in August 2000 to provide professional treatment for severe emergency patients in each region. The number of regional emergency medical centers has gradually increased over the years, and as of 2017, 39 centers are responding to emergency medical situations. These de velopments have contributed to the

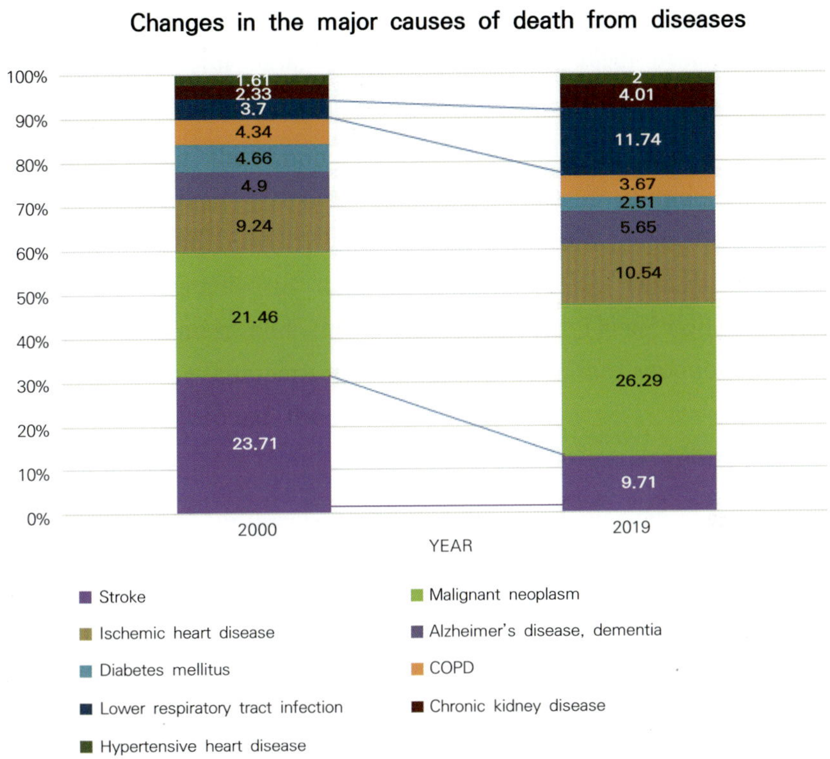

Figure 3-2. Changes in the major causes of death from diseases among the older adults in the domestic population (Global Health Estimate 2019: Deaths by Cause, Age, Sex, by Country and by Region, 2000-2019. Geneva, World Health Organization; 2020.) Abbreviation: COPD, chronic obstructive pulmonary disease.

decrease in deaths from stroke, despite the increase in the number of deaths among older adults due to the aging of the population and the increase in life expectancy.

The population of Korea is rapidly aging due to increased life expectancy and decreased birth rates. As a result, the number of deaths among older adults aged 70 or older increased more than 2.5 times in 2019 compared to 2000 [Ministry of Health and Welfare, 2019]. Malignant neoplasm has become the number one cause of death, accounting for more than a quarter of all causes of death. The number of deaths due to lower respiratory tract infections has increased five-fold in 20 years, and the percentage of deaths caused by lower respiratory tract infections has increased by about 3 times, making it the second leading cause of death among older adults in 2019. (Figure 3-2) Dementia, including Alzheimer's disease, for which old age is a representative risk factor, is also steadily increasing as a cause of death.

Ischemic heart disease is also a significant cause of death in Korea. Therefore, managing chronic illnesses, such as hypertension, diabetes mellitus, and hyperlipidemia, is crucial. Additionally, treating metabolic syndrome, such as obesity, by improving Western eating habits and reducing sedentary lifestyles is an essential health task [Nelson, ME, *et al.*, 2007]. Chronic disease management and lifestyle improvements are also crucial in reducing the steadily increasing number of chronic kidney disease and hypertensive heart disease deaths. Fortunately, the proportion of diabetes mellitus-related deaths is gradually decreasing, likely due to increased awareness of chronic diseases and improved medical access, leading to better diabetes mellitus control rates.

Changes in the Major High Disease Burden Diseases Among Older Adults

The term 'disability' refers to a state of functional limitation, and the number of years of healthy life lost due to this state is quantified using a metric called the Disability-Adjusted Life Year (DALY). The DALY was developed in the 1990s and is a widely used measure of disease burden, regularly published by the World

Health Organization. While many diseases that cause death also result in disability, DALY analysis can identify conditions that cause functional limitations without directly impacting lifespan.

Changes in the major high disease burden diseases worldwide

Based on data from the World Health Organization, we identified changes in diseases with high disease burdens among older adults worldwide. (Table 3-2)

Like the major causes of death, ischemic heart disease is the primary cause of disease burden [Park K *et al.*, 2021]. Ischemic heart disease occurs when the heart is not adequately supplied with nutrients and oxygen during times of increased demand, such as during exercise or physical labor. This can cause chest pain and restrict movement or work. In particular, myocardial infarction commonly causes heart failure, which is a condition where the pumping function of the heart is reduced because the part of the cardiac muscle where the infarction occurred is not functioning properly. The main symptom of heart failure is shortness of breath. When heart failure worsens, patients complain of shortness of breath even at rest, which makes it difficult to carry out daily activities.

Malignant neoplasm and stroke are the leading causes of death among older adults and also have a very high disease burden [Park K *et al.*, 2021]. As malignant neoplasm progresses, the symptoms vary depending on the primary site but often include pain, difficulty eating, shortness of breath, and changes in mental status, making daily life difficult. Stroke is known to cause various symptoms such as hemiplegia, facial paralysis, and dysarthria, which depend on the location and size of the affected brain tissue, often leading to disability.

Table 3-2. **Changes in the top 10 high disease burden diseases among older adults worldwide** (Global Health Estimate 2019: Disease burden by Cause, Age, Sex, by Country and Region, 2000-2019. Geneva, World Health Organization; 2020.) Abbreviation: COPD, chronic obstructive pulmonary disease.

Ranking	2000	2010	2015	2019	Note
1	Ischemic heart disease	Ischemic heart disease	Ischemic heart disease	Ischemic heart disease	
2	Stroke	Stroke	Malignant neoplasm	Malignant neoplasm	
3	Malignant neoplasm	Malignant neoplasm	Stroke	Stroke	
4	COPD	COPD	COPD	COPD	
5	Diabetes mellitus	Alzheimer's disease, dementia	Alzheimer's disease, dementia	Alzheimer's disease, dementia	
6	Lower respiratory tract infection	Diabetes mellitus	Diabetes mellitus	Diabetes mellitus	
7	Diarrheal disease	Lower respiratory tract infection	Lower respiratory tract infection	Lower respiratory tract infection	
8	Alzheimer's disease, dementia	Hearing loss	Hearing loss	Hearing loss	
9	Hearing loss	Diarrheal disease	Chronic kidney disease	Chronic kidney disease	
10	Hypertensive heart disease	Chronic kidney disease	Hypertensive heart disease	Fall	

As pulmonary function declines severely, people with COPD may experience severe respiratory distress, reducing exercise capacity, muscle weakness, and weight loss [Park K *et al.*, 2021]. As a result, this can significantly impact their daily life, as they may be frequently hospitalized due to acute exacerbations and require respiratory support devices at home. Unfortunately, for those who have been living with COPD for a long time, these restrictions can become a regular part of their life.

In 2019, dementia, including Alzheimer's disease, caused a significant increase in disease burden compared to 2000, accounting for more than 5% of the total disease burden among older adults [Park K *et al.*, 2021]. Alzheimer's disease, a common form of dementia, results in the gradual loss of all daily living functions and the development of various behavioral and psychological symptoms, such as delusions, hallucinations, and increased aggression. These symptoms often occur together, leading to a significant burden of care.

Diabetes mellitus is a major cause of death, accounting for a large proportion of the disease burden [Korean Diabetes Association, 2020]. Treatment of diabetes mellitus, including the use of insulin, requires considerable effort, and complications of the disease can result in various functional limitations. For instance, diabetic retinopathy may lead to blindness, diabetic nephropathy may necessitate regular dialysis treatment, and diabetic neuropathy may cause numbness and pain in the hands and feet. Considering that the burden of diseases such as chronic kidney disease and hypertensive heart disease is gradually increasing, managing chronic diseases is essential for reducing the overall disease burden.

Although hearing loss and falls are not among the top 10 leading causes of death in 2019, they are among the top 10 diseases with a high disease burden. Age-related deafness, also known as senile deafness, is the most common sensory abnormality associated with aging, and its prevalence increases rapidly with age. Approximately 40% of people over 70 years old have presbycusis, and when hearing loss occurs, communication becomes difficult, leading to various problems in daily life. Unfortunately, drug treatment cannot improve or restore age-related hearing loss. However, early detection and the use of hearing aids can help patients better adapt to daily life. Falls are also a prevalent health issue that increases in incidence with age, and the occurrence of injuries such as fractures is a significant problem. Even if no physical harm occurs, fear of falling can reduce mobility in older adults. Therefore, preventing falls is essential, and measures such as exercise and environmental modifications can help reduce the risk of falls in older adults.

Changes in the major high disease burden diseases in the domestic population

In Korea, diseases with a high disease burden show similar changes to those of major causes of death. In 2000, stroke was the disease with the highest burden among older adults, and this was also the case in other upper-middle-income countries. However, by 2019, malignant neoplasm had become the top disease with a high burden of disease in Korea, as it is in high-income countries. Meanwhile, lower respiratory tract infections have been increasing rapidly among older adults and became the second leading cause of death in 2019, leading to a steady increase in their disease burden. (Figure 3-3)

As the population is aging rapidly, the disease burden of dementia and hearing loss, which is closely related to age, is steadily increasing. In contrast, the burden of diabetes mellitus seems to be gradually decreasing due to reduced complications caused by improved control rates [Korean Diabetes Association, 2020]. Recent data from the Korea National Health and Nutrition Examination Survey showed that the diabetes mellitus control rate among people aged 65 or older has increased by over 5% in the past five years. However, diabetes mellitus remains a significant health concern, and ongoing attention and efforts are necessary to improve control rates and reduce the disease burden.

In Korea, arthritis is a disease with a high disease burden among older adults. Degenerative arthritis is a representative form of the disease caused by aging-related degenerative changes in articular cartilage, which is why most patients are older adults. Due to the progressive nature of the disease, it is crucial to prevent rapid progression of joint damage and improve patients' quality of life by reducing pain and increasing range of motion. Weight loss can be beneficial for overweight patients, while avoiding repetitive tasks and using assistive devices like canes can reduce joint stress.

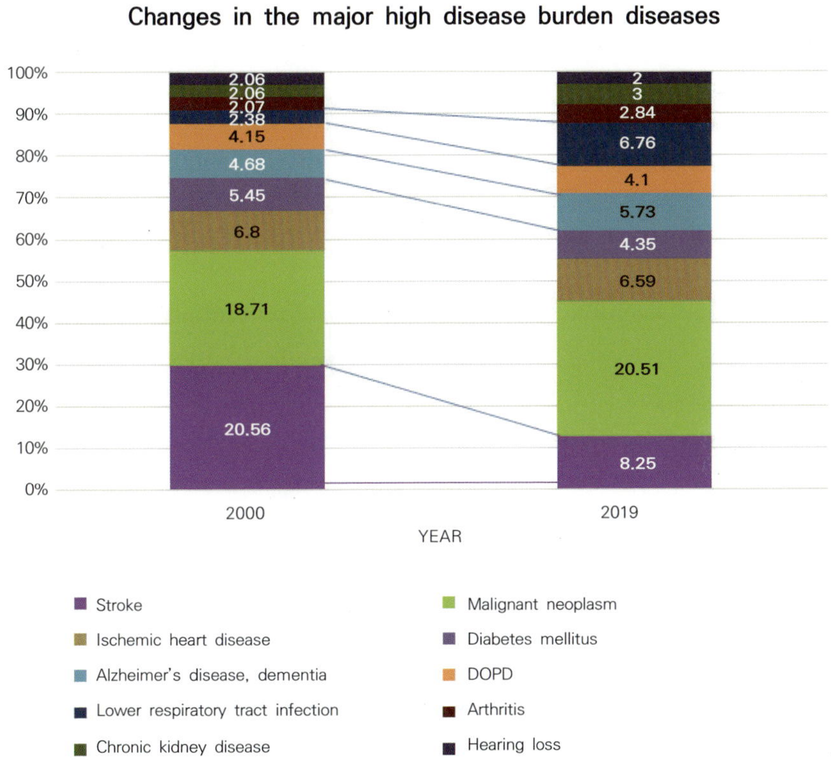

Figure 3-3. Changes in the major high disease burden diseases among the older adults in the domestic population (Global Health Estimate 2019: Disease burden by Cause, Age, Sex, by Country and by Region, 2000-2019. Geneva, World Health Organization; 2020.) Abbreviation: COPD, chronic obstructive pulmonary disease.

Although falls and back pain are not currently among the top 10 diseases in terms of burden, they are likely to become more prevalent in the near future based on increasing trends. Falls, which mainly affect older adults, are on the rise due to the growing older population. In 2015, the Evidence-based Guideline for Fall Prevention was established in Korea to address this issue. The guideline includes recommendations for fall prevention, evaluation and intervention, gait and balance assessment, and fall prevention exercises. Spinal pain, including back pain, is a significant health concern in developed countries like the United States and Japan, and can greatly impact function and quality of life. Therefore, more attention is needed to address this issue.

Life Principles to Extend a Healthy Lifespan

Extending healthy lifespan has become a more important issue than simply extending lifespan, as people aim to live a longer life free from disease and disability. In Korea, it is reported that people suffer from diseases for more than 15 years of their lives, highlighting the importance of extending healthy lifespan. To achieve this, it is essential to prevent the major diseases mentioned above, minimize disability, and maintain independent function as much as possible by effectively managing them. Instead of coping with each disease individually, it is wiser to follow healthy living principles to maintain good health [Nelson ME, *et al.*, 2007]. There are three options to achieve this:

(1) It is necessary to maintain a healthy lifestyle to prevent disease.
(2) It is important to detect diseases at an early stage through regular checkups and to treat those diseases immediately.
(3) It is essential to manage chronic diseases thoroughly.

Summary

Population aging is a global phenomenon, but Korea is experiencing an unusually rapid transition into a super-aged society. The rapid increase in the aging population inevitably leads to a significant rise in socio-economic burdens, especially in medical expenses. In 2017, medical expenses for adults 65 years or older accounted for KRW 27.6 trillion out of the total KRW 69.3 trillion in medical expenses covered by health insurance, representing 40% of the total. The cost of care is also increasing as the proportion of older people living alone continues to rise. As a result, the social burden on older adults is increasing in various ways. Given the inevitability of population aging, it is essential to focus on efforts towards healthy aging as a critical task, not only for the quality of life of the older population but also for socioeconomic reasons.

References

- Department of Internal Medicine, College of Medicine, Seoul National University, SNUH manual of medicine, 4th edition, Korea Medicine, 2018.
- Howard M. Fillit *et al.* Brocklehurst's Textbook of Geriatric Medicine and Gerontology, 8th Edition, Elsevier, 2016.
- Kontis V, Bennett JE, Mathers CD, Li G, Foreman K, Ezzati M. Future life expectancy in 35 industrialised countries: projections with a Bayesian model ensemble. Lancet (London, England). 2017;389(10076):1323-1335.
- Korea Centers for Disease Control and Prevention National Health Information Portal (http://health.kdca.go.kr/)
- Korean Diabetes Association, Diabetes fact sheet in Korea 2020.
- Park K *et al.* Korean centenarians: 20 years of change. Koonja Publishing Inc., 2021.
- Ministry of Health and Welfare, 2019 National Health Statistics.
- Nelson ME, Rejeski WJ, Blair SN, Duncan PW, Judge JO, King AC, *et al.* Physical activity and public health in older adults: recommendation from the American College of Sports Medicine and the American Heart Association. Circulation. 2007;116(9):1094-1105.
- Seoul National University Bundang Hospital Senior Medical Center, Treatment Encyclopedia for the older adults, 1st edition, RH Korea, 2021.
- Seoul National University Hospital Medical Information (http://www.snuh.org/)
- The Korean Geriatrics Society, Geriatrics fact sheet 2018.
- The Korean Geriatrics Society, Textbook of Geriatric Medicine, 3rd edition, Beommun Education, 2015.
- The Korean Society of Hypertension, Korea Hypertension fact sheet 2020.

PART II

CHANGES IN FAMILY AND SOCIAL WELFARE SYSTEM FOR OLDER PEOPLE IN KOREA

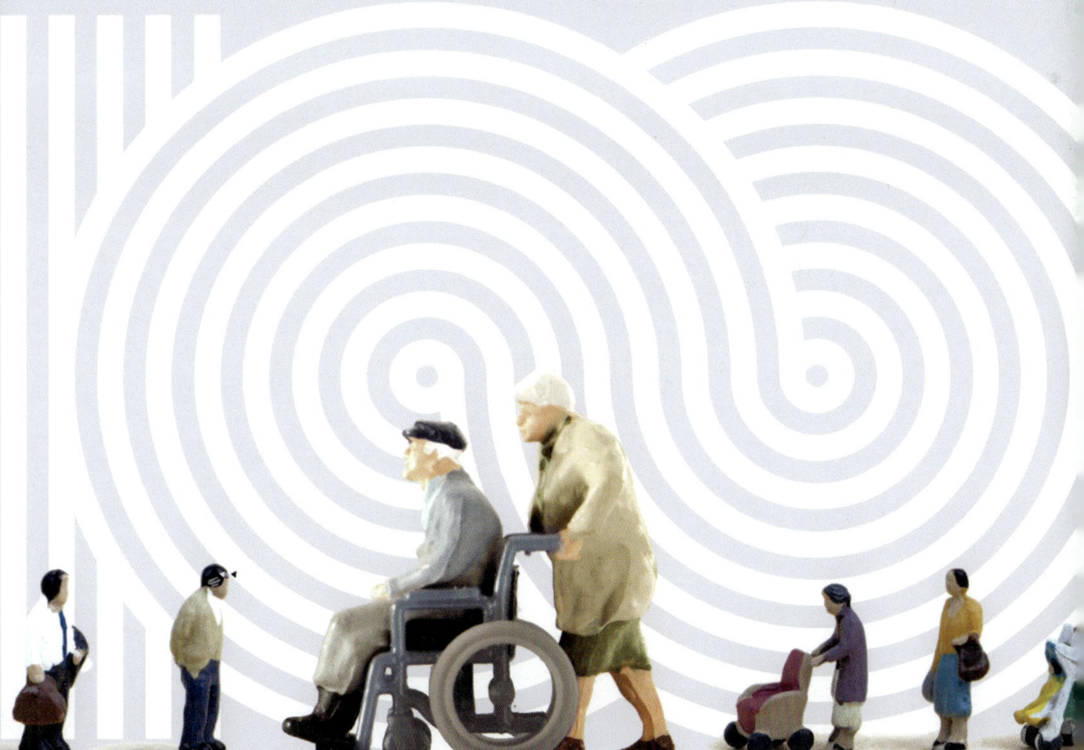

Chapter 04

Changes in the Care and Family Systems of Korean Centenarians

Jeonghwa Lee

A person living for more than a century can be said to be a hero in the sense that this is the result of overcoming various challenges and difficulties in life. Although many years have passed since Korea became an aging society in 2000 and there has been a rapid increase in the number of super-aged people (aged 100 and older), there has been little in-depth understanding of who they are and their quality of life.

The first study on centenarian families in Korea was conducted in the early 2000s [Han GH, 2002]. In this study, the family history and family relationship dynamics of Korean centenarians were identified, and the quality of life of centenarians with respect to their families was investigated. The quality of life of centenarians was mainly determined by their health, economic conditions, and relationships with caregivers. This is due in large part to the fact that family is a key factor in determining the quality of life of centenarians in Korea. Traditionally, the most important characteristics in Korean family relationships involve a strong son-centered and eldest son-centered life. This often resulted in problems when it comes to support for the family of the eldest son, difficulties in supporting daughters, and a poor quality of life for the elderly living alone. The interpretation of parental longevity generally reflects the long-standing relationship history and the quality of family relationships between centenarians and their children. In families with good generational relationships, the longevity of parents is interpreted positively. Meanwhile, families with poor generational relationships and high support burdens when it comes to dependents think very negatively about the longevity of centenarians. According to this study, there should be a fairer support system to improve the quality of life of centenarians and their families than the eldest son-centered support norms. In addition, it was concluded that social policy support was urgently needed.

Further research on centenarians and their families in Korea was conducted in 2018 and 2022. The 2018 study, which was the second study on Korean centenarians and their families, focused on the changes in the lives of centenarians between 2001 and 2018[Lee J *et al.*, 2021: Park K *et al.*, 2021]. In particular, this study took a special interest in the changes in family caregiving and interactions with the community. The 2022 study, the third study on Korean centenarians and their families, focused on quality of life and caregiving. In particular, the positive and negative effects of the self-care, family-provided care, and public care of centenarians were explored.

By examining the results of earlier Korean centenarian studies, this study examines how the life of centenarians has changed and what social changes are behind these differences. In addition, it sheds new light on the roles of family, community, and public policy in the lives of centenarians.

Research Methods

These studies were conducted in the Korean Longevity Belt (Gurye, Goksung, Sunchang and Damyang counties) in the provinces of North Cholla and South Cholla. This region has a relatively high percentage of the oldest-old. Since the number of centenarians is limited, this study was expanded to include seniors over the age of 95(near-centenarians). This study was conducted in cooperation with the governing administrations for the counties under study. Public officers provided guidance and introductions to the oldest-old and their caregivers.

This study was based on the results of surveys conducted in 2018 and 2022. In 2018, there were 53 near-centenarians and 45 centenarians in the Korean Longevity Belt. From a total of 98 cases, 62 centenarians and their caregivers were interviewed. In 2022, there were 79 near-centenarians and centenarians in that same area. Among them, 74 centenarians and their caregivers were interviewed. The qualitative and phenomenological surveys included in-depth interviews and observations using semi-structured questionnaires administered to the elderly, their families, care providers, and nursing home staff.

Four researchers in two teams visited residences to conduct investigations and record interviews. They also obtained informed consent after explaining the purpose of the study and confidentiality. The responses were transcribed verbatim for analysis and to elicit a number of emerging themes from interviews. The researchers analyzed the data by excluding prejudice through regular meetings and by checking interviews and field notes in a neutral way.

Changes in the Living Arrangements of Korean Centenarians and Their Interactions with Family and Community

What are some of the changes in the lives of centenarians?

It can be seen that there have been many changes in the lives of centenarians. Above all, the overall level of education has increased. The number of centenarians who can read Hangul (the Korean alphabet) has increased from 13% to 36%, and the number of respondents who answered that their subjective living standards were above average increased from 33% to 44.5%. In fact, it can be observed that the number of centenarians who manage their own lives has increased and that the economic situation of this group as a whole has significantly improved when compared to the past.

Who do they live with, and who cares for them?

Older people in Korea are highly dependent on their families due largely to the fact that Korea is a blood-centered, family-oriented society. As a result, the meaning of family in old age is highly significant. For the most part, the centenarians in this study had many children who became a source of support. They had an average of 4.6 living adult children. Twenty years ago, there were only two surviving adult children because their lifespan was not long. Compared to the past, more support resources are available for centenarians.

A number of things can be learned by looking at the living arrangements of the oldest-old. In 2001, 100% of them lived in their own home, and the percentage of people living alone was only 12%. However, by 2018, 51% of this group lived with their families, 31% lived alone, and 17% lived in nursing homes. This shows a large change in terms of living arrangements. This change is a result of changes in the structure of Korean caregiving. In particular, the number of older people living in nursing homes and hospitals has increased. This is due to the long-term care insurance system implemented in 2008. This insurance system has had a significant effect on the increased acceptance rate of the elderly into long-term care facilities.

The greatest change in terms of families is the fact that when compared with 2001, the number of older people living with their daughter-in-law decreased by one-third. In the past, the eldest son and the eldest daughter-in-law were the primary caregivers in Korea. Recently, this has changed to a more equitable method of sharing responsibilities among children. This change is related to an

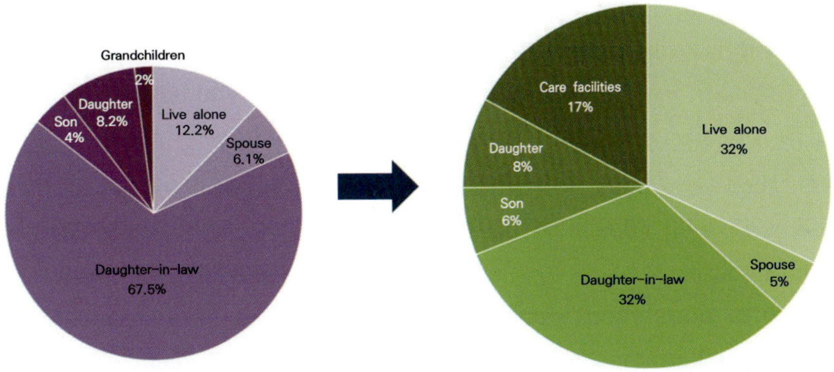

〈Living Arrangements in 2001〉

- Daughter-in-law 67.5%
- Son and daughters 12.2%
- Live alone 12.2%
- Care facilities 0%

〈Living Arrangements in 2018〉

- Daughter-in-law 32%
- Son and daughters 14%
- Live alone 32%
- Care facilities 17%

Figure 4-1. Changes in living arrangements between 2001 and 2018

increase in family dissolutions due to divorce or the death of adult children, and the inclusion of women in the labor market since they were primarily responsible for caregiving in the past. These findings show a weakening of the caregiving norm with respect to the eldest son. These days, siblings take turns caring for parents and it is common for the caregiver to be the third/or youngest son. In addition, sons participate in taking care of their elderly parents considerably more than in 2001. Sons are willing to participate in their parents' bathing, feeding, and dressing. Daughters supporting behavior has also increased. There are not many daughters living together with their parents. However, they take care of their elderly parents as much as their sons.

Family Interactions with Korean Centenarians Based on Residence Type

This study examines three different residence types and shows that there are differences in the characteristics of interactions with family members based on the residence type. The three types of residences examined in this study are centenarians living with family members, centenarians living alone, and centenarians living in long-term care facilities.

The first group of centenarians examined in this study included those living with family members. In terms of family cohabitation, there have been cases where adult children have lived with their parents all their lives. However, there have been many cases where adult children have moved back to their hometowns to be with their parents and where elderly parents have returned to their hometowns to be with their children. Elderly parents were found to be very afraid of going to nursing homes far away from their families. It was also found that some of the elderly parents in this study had sicker adult children than they were themselves. It also it turns out that brothers sometimes share the caregiving burden when they have good sibling relationships. They often resent this caregiving burden if the relationships are not that strong.

The second group of centenarians under study included those living alone. 20 (32%) of the participants of this study were found to be living alone. It was determined that the lives of centenarians living alone are quite different from the past. The centenarians living alone were physically healthier and more cognitive than the respondents in other living arrangements. In the past, not many centenarians lived alone, and their quality of life was very poor. In addition, no male centenarians lived alone in the earlier study. However, it has been estimated that a third of the older male population lives alone. These results explain why there are mechanisms in place for the oldest-old to live alone. The first of these mechanisms is family support, where adult children visit or call their parents at least once a week. There is also formal and institutional support. Health care workers visit older people every day and are equipped with lunch delivery and emergency phone services. In addition, the government provides a basic old-age pension. There is also support from the community. Older people in Korea usually have a place where they can gather every day, meet their neighbors, and share their food to prevent them from being lonely.

The third and final group of centenarians was made up of those living in long-term care facilities (nursing homes). 10 (17%) of the participants were found to be living in such facilities. Most of them require a wheelchair, mobility assistance, and diapers. The centenarians living in care facilities were generally not isolated since their children

	N(%)	Remarks	
Care facilities	10(14.3)	Nursing home 9 cases Nursing hospital 1 case	Care facilities
Adult day care center	2(2.9)		Live alone & Live with family
Home health care service/Home health care service by family members	30(42.9)	Home health care service by daughter-in-law 1 case	
Solitary Elderly Care Manager	3(4.3)		
Others	9(12.9)	Bathing service Food delivery service	
None	16(22.9)		
Total	70(100%)		

※ Some people are using more than one service.

Figure 4-2. Increase of systematic care services use in 2018

visited them. Some of these children visit frequently. When visitations were not frequent, they occurred at least once every few months. In addition to nursing homes, elderly daycare centers have recently emerged as an alternative. Due to traditional Confucian ideas, there is a stigma associated with having parents in nursing homes. These daycare centers are emerging as an alternative to lower the emotional barriers in the minds of parents and adult children when it comes to entering elderly care facilities.

The Standard of Living, Quality of Life, and Type of Caregiving of Centenarians

Standard of living of centenarians

The standard of living of centenarians was divided into housing, economic status, and independence, and various levels were identified. Researchers made direct observations while conducting surveys and evaluated the level of housing, economic status, and independence. Three levels, “upper,” “middle,” and “lower,” were identified while referring to data provided in the form of research notes, photos, and transcriptions. To increase the reliability of the living standard evaluations, four researchers engaged in extensive discussion over several hours while looking at the data together.

In terms of the housing level of centenarians, 45.9% (34 people) of the total were evaluated to be “middle”, followed by 29.7% (22 people) at “upper”, and 24.3% (18 people) at “lower.” For the economic status level, the proportion of “middle” was the highest at 44.6% (33 people), followed by “lower” at 28.4% (21 people), and “upper” at 27.0% (20 people). When it comes to the independence level of centenarians, “upper” was the highest at 37.8% (28 people) of the total, followed by “middle” at 33.8% (25 people), and “lower” at 28.4% (21 people). Overall, the housing and economic levels of centenarians were shown to be “middle’, while the level of centenarian independence was shown to be relatively high.

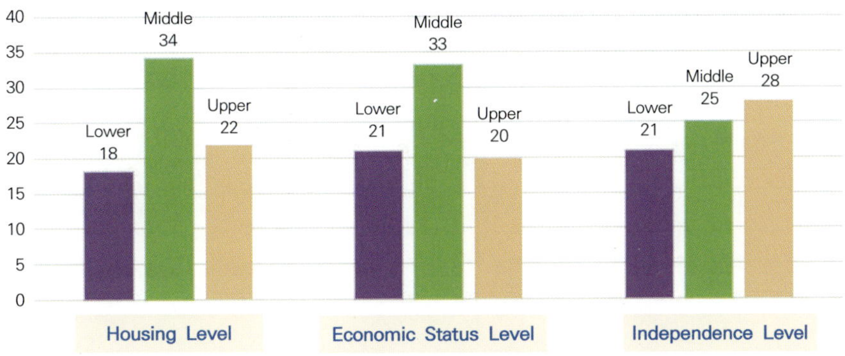

Figure 4-3. Standard of living : Housing, economic status, and independence level

Quality of life of centenarians

To understand the quality of life of centenarians, 100 points were given to a level where it was not overly inconvenient for centenarians to maintain their daily life through an overall evaluation of their level of housing, economy, and independence as well as support. In other words, 100 points in terms of quality of life were set at a level that would not make daily life very uncomfortable, even if it is not the best condition for living. The quality of life scores was given in decrements of 10 points where the lower the quality of life score, the more difficult it was for a person to maintain their daily life.

The quality of life of centenarians was 100 points for 37 people (50%), 90 points for 5 people (6.8%), 80 points for 14 people (18.9%), 70 points for 12 people (16.2%), 60 points for 5 people (6.8%), and 50 points for 1 person (1.4%). The average quality of life for centenarians was 87.3, with a standard deviation (SD) of 14.6. When a quality of life score of fewer than 70 points is classified as "low," 80 to 90 points are classified as "medium," and 100 points is classified as "high," it can be interpreted that about half

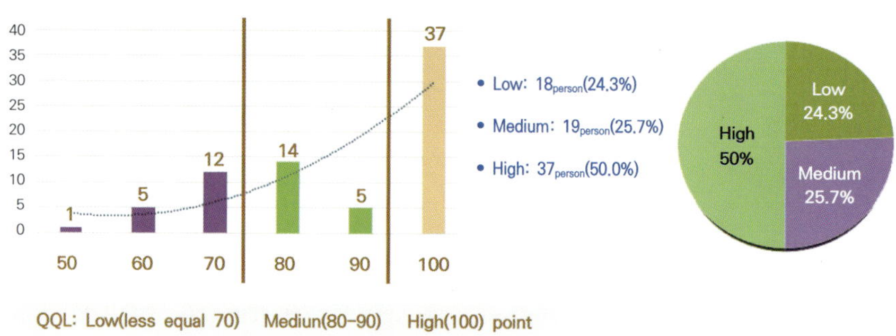

Figure 4-4. Quality of life of centenarians

of centenarians have no major inconvenience in maintaining their daily lives.

Types of caregiving for centenarians

The effects of caregiving status on the quality of life of centenarians were identified. The impacts of self-care, family provided-care, and public care on the quality of life of centenarians in terms of housing, economy, and independence were examined. To this end, the ratio of self-care, family provided-care, and public care was calculated and scored with reference to the quality of life score of centenarians. In other words, scores were given in each area based on the degree of self-care, the degree of support from family members (such as spouses, children, and grandchildren), and the degree of public support services provided by state or local governments. In other words, self-care, family provided-care, and public-care scores were allocated to the quality of life scores.

Self-care, family provided-care, and public-care of centenarians

The overall quality of life scores of centenarians ranged from a minimum of 50 points to a maximum of 100 points, with an average score of 87.3 (SD=14.6). These scores indicate that a person is maintaining their daily life at a level that is somewhat but not overly uncomfortable. As a result of allocating centenarians' self-care, family provided-care, and public-care scores based on their quality of life score, the average self-care (range: 0 to 80) was 40.2 (SD=18.2), the average family provided-care (range: 0 to 80) was 33.0 (SD=15.3), and the average public-care (range: 0 to 40) was 14.1 (SD=11.5). The average support gap, which is not filled by self, family

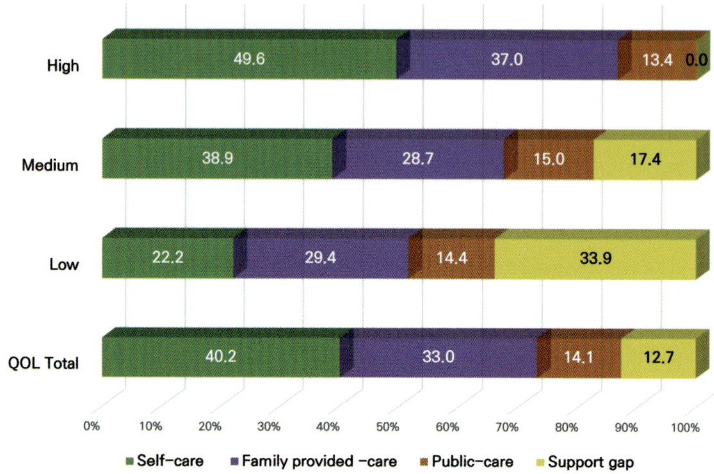

Figure 4-5. Quality of life and self-care / family provided-care / public care

provided, and public care, was 12.7 (SD=14.6). Centenarians had the highest scores when engaging in self-care, followed by those receiving family provided-care. From these results, it can be seen that to maintain the daily life of centenarians without undue difficulty, a plan is needed to reduce the average support gap of 12.7 points.

The caregiving types of centenarians were largely divided into specific area-centered, balanced, and mixed types. The specific area-centered types are self-care-centered, family provided-care-centered, and public-care-centered, while the balanced type is a harmonious self/family provided/public care ratio. The mixed type is a type of caregiving supported by a mixture of self, family provided, and public care, which can be divided into a self/family provided care mixed type, a self/public care mixed type, and a family provided/public care mixed type. Among these types of caregiving for elderly people, 45.9% were self-care-centered, followed by 27.0% family provided-care-centered, 9.5% balanced care, 8.1% self/family provided-care mixed, 4.1% family provoded/public-care mixed, 2.7% public care-centered, and 2.7% self/public care mixed

Most of the centenarians in this study had self-care-centered care, leading to a self-directed life. The next most common type of care is the family provided-care-centered type, where adult children mainly supported centenarians to minimize inconvenience. Centenarians, who had a high quality of life, mainly had a high level of self-care. They maintained a constant level of health, and took the initiative in their daily lives, such as eating, fieldwork, bathing, and grooming. Centenarian self-care level was closely linked to the level of health, since appropriate activities are needed to maintain a certain level of health. It was found that confidence in the activities and the conditions for these activities had an important effect on centenarian health, longevity, and high cognitive functioning. However, it was found that if centenarians lack self-care capabilities, their quality of life can be kept high when family provided and public care are organically linked.

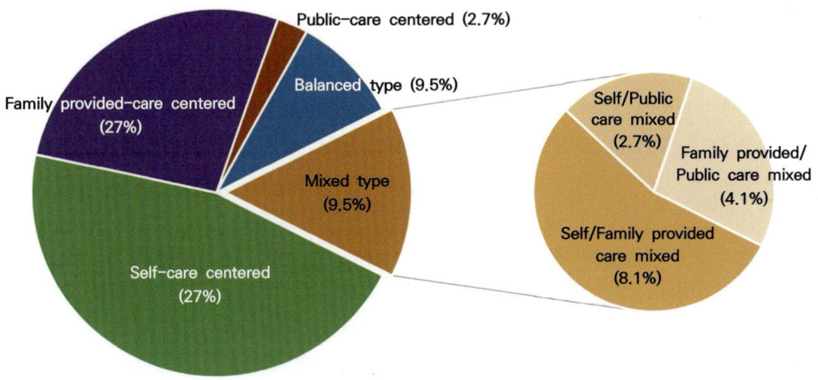

Figure 4-6. The caregiving type

Summary

In recent years, the family structures and family interactions of centenarians in Korea have undergone dramatic changes. The traditional Korean family norm (son-centered, especially the eldest son and daughter-in-law-centered) has weakened. Any adult children who can afford to care for their elderly parents, regardless of birth order or gender, can be caregivers. Despite these changes in caregiving norms and an increase in the family dissolution of adult children, 83% of the centenarians still live in their community. This is due in large part to the creation of long-term care insurance and home health care services. In addition, centenarians who live alone or in care facilities have at least one adult child with whom they have regular contact. Meanwhile, centenarians as a whole have an average of 4.6 living children. However, in the future, older adults will have fewer children, which means there will be limited caregiving resources. Even if family caregiving shifts to community caregiving, emotional care and interaction with family will still be keys to the quality of life of older adults. Therefore, systematic cooperation between families and communities has become increasingly important. Such cooperation also makes it possible for older adults to live in their community for a longer time.

In addition, in Korean society, which will soon become a super-aged society, thinking about the quality of life of centenarians is a way to prepare for the future of society. Providing appropriate care and living environments for the super-aged is a very important topic in Korean society. In terms of the support for centenarians, this study emphasized a balance between self-care, family provided-care, and public-care. In this study, the centenarians who had a high quality of life, generally had a high level of self-care. It was found that the confidence and surrounding environments of centenarians in their activities have an important effect on their health, longevity, and high cognitive functioning. The complex needs of the people living in centenarian communities and their families vary. These needs include economic problems, housing problems, nutrition problems, and family care burdens. The most functional and dynamic model that has been found in the field is "a model in which self-care, family provided-care, and public-care are harmonized so it is not inconvenient to carry on in daily life."

The most important resource in self-care is the self-care competency of hundred-year-olds. To maintain the self-care capabilities of centenarians, strategic intervention activities are needed to provide healthcare-related information on meal management, walking, or gymnastics, and to encourage and support the elderly to maintain their own health.

For family provided-care to function properly, it is necessary to provide information on the resources and public facilities that families can use when taking care of hundred-year-olds. Since most of the adult children of centenarians are also elderly, the supporters who provide care for the oldest-old also need services to receive treatment and care.

In terms of public-care, case management for centenarians will become more important. The overall care culture and care systems in Korean society need to be actively prepared so that centenarians can face a dignified old age in the final stage of life.

In a super-aged society, a well-established care system for centenarians will enable AIP (Aging in Place) so that older people can face a dignified retirement. Above all, it is necessary to change the perception that the super-aged are lethargic and weak. It should be emphasized that they are often capable of self-management and can lead their own lives. In addition, multidisciplinary research and policy development should be further activated so that more centenarians can manage their daily lives independently.

References

- Han GH. Family relationships and quality of life of Korean centenarians. In Park SC. (Eds.) Korean centenarian study. Seoul: Seoul National University Press, 2002.
- Lee J, Oh YE, Lee B. A Qualitative Study on the living arrangements and life of Korean centenarians. Family and Culture. 2021;33(3):102-142.
- Park K *et al*. Korean centenarians: 20 years of change. Koonja Publishing Inc., 2021.

Chapter 05

Changes in the Social Welfare System for Older Adults in Korea

Kichae Min

Introduction

At the national level, there are virtually no social welfare systems for long-lived seniors. In this chapter, we will look at the changes in the social welfare system for older adults over the past 60 years from the 1960s to the 2020s. To this end, we examine changes in the Social Welfare Act for older adults from a diachronic perspective and understand changes in the old-age income security system and social welfare services for older adults. By understanding the historical process of change, we explore the direction of senior welfare policies for centenarians.

Changes in Social Welfare System for Older Adults in 60 Years: From the 1960s to the 2020s

1960s to 1970s : the birth of the care service for older adults in need of care

Korea's welfare system for older adults in a modern sense can be found in the 「Joseon Relief Order」 enacted in 1944. Article 1 ① of the 「Joseon Relief Order」, which was only a tool of governance during colonial rule, stipulates that "If the following persons are unable to live due to poverty, relief is provided according to this order", and 'older adults aged 65 years or older' are included. In addition, subsidies for livelihood, medical care, midwifery, and occupation assistance have been presented. The legal content of the 「Joseon Relief Order」 was succeeded by the 「Livelihood Protection Law」 enacted in 1961. When historically understanding the welfare system for older adults, it can be said that it was a period of relief work for older adults in need of care. At that time, the residual care service for older adults without family to take care of them was introduced.

1980s : Changes from care to welfare for older adults

With the introduction of the 「Welfare of Senior Citizens Act」 (enacted in 1981), it was announced that the subject of care for older adults would shift from the family to society. The legal basis for implementing welfare services for older adults was prepared, and the existing care service for older adults was converted into welfare services for older adults. In short, 'socialization of caring' has sprouted in the welfare of older adults. However, since welfare was still subordinated to economic growth, welfare for older adults was almost ignored at the social level.

1990s : Expansion of welfare for older adults

Welfare services for older adults at home, which allow people to use welfare services while living in the community rather than facilities, have been expanded. At this time, the subject of the supply of welfare services for older adults was expanded to the private sector. In 1997, the 「Welfare of Senior Citizens Act」 was amended to guarantee income security and medical care for older adults. In particular, the income security system was introduced in 1989, focusing on the payment of old age allowance for low-income older adults over 65 years of age. It was a time when the welfare system for older adults was gradually expanding.

2000s : Expansion of socialization of care

The coverage and the contents of benefits for older adults were expanded. Meal delivery service for low-income older adults at home with mobility difficulties started in 2000, and is currently implemented at senior welfare centers across the country. A provision related to the prohibition of elder abuse was newly established in the 「Welfare of Senior Citizens Act」. The job project for older adults started in 2004. With the enactment of the 「Long-Term Care Insurance Act」 in 2007, the long-term care supply infrastructure was expanded, and the socialization of care for older adults based on insurance finance began in earnest. In addition, with the enactment of the 「Basic Senior Pensions Act」 in 2007, the state responsibility of poverty for older adults was emphasized.

2010s : Diversification of welfare for older adults

Welfare services for older adults have diversified. Laws and policies related to housing, dementia, leisure, transportation/movement services, and support for senior citizens associations were introduced. It was a time when welfare for older adults was diversified by widely socializing the special needs of older adults without narrowing it down to income and health.

2020s : Consolidation of the welfare system for older adults

Currently, welfare for older adults in Korea is being consolidated. The welfare system for older adults related to housing, medical care, nursing, dementia, caring, employment, and leisure activities for older adults is settling down. Various systems for the needs of older adults have been continuously developed, and various infrastructures are also expanding. Recently, it has been expanding to community care that pursues an integrated care model.

Changes in the Social Welfare Act for Older Adults

Over the past 60 years, the welfare system for older adults in Korea has had a 'history of institutional expansion' to address the social risks of senescence. The basis for this is the expansion of welfare acts for older adults. In the past, the comprehensiveness of the welfare system for older adults was very small. In short, there was a lack of institutions to respond to social risks.

Before 2000, at the level of the social insurance laws, the 「National Pension Act」(1973) was enacted, but it was ineffective, and the actual implementation of the system began in 1988. The 「National Health Insurance Act」(1963) also began as a voluntary application rather than a compulsory one. The national health security system was established by integrated operation as a single insurer. Next, from the perspective of public assistance laws, except for the 「National Basic Living Security Act」(1961) and the 「Medical Benefit Act」, the social assistance system for vulnerable older adults with low income was insignificant. Lastly, regarding social service laws, finding legislation related to social services other than a few key acts is challenging. These include the 「Welfare of Senior Citizens Act」(1981), the 「Lifelong Education Act」(1982), and the 「Act on Prohibition of Age Discrimination in Employment and Elderly Employment Promotion」(1991).

In 2000, entering the era of the welfare state, various social security laws were enacted. The welfare sector for older adults was no exception. Since 2000, various welfare laws for older adults have been enacted in all areas of social insurance, public assistance, and social services. From the perspective of the Basic Law, it is necessary to pay attention to the enactment of the 「Framework Act on Low Birth Rate in an Aging Society」 in 2005. With the enactment of the law, it can be evaluated that it contributed to the formation of a consensus that the national crisis of 'low birth and population aging' was recognized and that a response was necessary. In particular, it is meaningful in that it has established and evaluated the master plan 'Basic Plan for Low Fertility and Aging Society' four times through the Act. From the perspective of social insurance laws, the 「Long-Term Care Insurance Act」 was enacted in 2007, establishing the framework of the five major social insurance systems. With the introduction of long-term care insurance for older adults, it was able to receive evaluations such as socializing care, strengthening national responsibility of care burden, and weakening the stigma against the Confucian welfare state, which presupposes the sacrifice of women. Most notably, through the 「Basic Pension Act」 (2007), the basic pension scheme began to be paid on January 1, 2008. In 2007, the law was enacted, older adults' poverty rate in Korea was 44.6%, and about 1 out of 2 older adults were poor [OECD, 2013].

Changes in the Old-Age Income Security

Changes in the old-age income security system

The old-age income security system can be evaluated as 'a change from a formal multi-tier old-age income security system to a practical multi-tier old-age income security system' when comparing the pre-2000 and 2023 present(Figure 5-1). The old-age income security system before 2000 was formed in four tiers : old age allowance on the 0th tier, national pension on the 1st tier, lump sum retirement payment on the 2nd tier, private pension on the 3rd tier, and earned income on the 4th tier. The old age allowance on the 0th tier was targeted at the recipients of national basic livelihood security and low-income seniors, but compared to the current basic pension system, it is applied to a smaller number of recipients, and the benefit level is lower, so a dotted line indicates it. Also, a dotted line indicates retirement pay because there is a limit to defining it as a stable old-age income security since you receive a 'lump sum' rather than a 'pension' method.

The current old-age income security system consists of five tiers: basic pension on the 0th tier, national pension on the 1st tier, retirement pension on the 2nd tier, private pension on the 3rd tier, and earned income on the 4th tier. With the introduction of the 「Basic Pension Act」 in 2007 and the enactment of the 「Act on the Guarantee of Employees' Retirement Benefits」 in 2005, a multi-tier old-age security system was established.

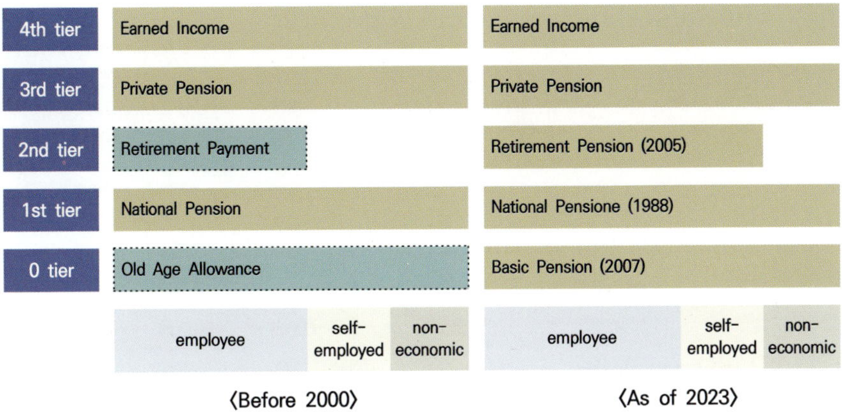

Figure 5-1. Changes in the old-age income security system in Korea: comparison between before 2000 and 2023

Changes in old-age income security scheme

Looking at the major changes, first of all, the old-age income security system for the purpose of basic livelihood security for older adults in difficult living has changed. The old age allowance changed to the basic old-age pension and from the basic old-age pension to the basic pension. The old age allowance, which had been paid to the subject to livelihood protection since 1991, was replaced with the old age allowance in July 1998. As of 2001, 715,108 people were eligible for support of the old age allowance, and the amount of support was 50,000 won for recipients of national basic livelihood security aged 80 or older. It was 40,000 won for those aged 65 to 79, and 30,000 won for low-income seniors who did not receive the National Basic Livelihood Security [Ministry of Health and Welfare, 2001]. The coverage was expanded in the process of reforming from old age benefit to old age allowance, and in the process of introducing the basic senior pension system and the basic pension system, it was greatly expanded to 70% of

Table 5-1. Number of insured persons: 1988~2023

(2023.1.31., unit: persons)

	Total number of insured Persons	Workplace-based insured persons	Individually insured persons	Voluntarily insured persons	Voluntarily & continuously insured persons
1988.12.31.	4,432,695	4,431,039	-	1,370	286
1992.12.31.	5,021,159	4,977,441	-	32,238	11,480
1995.12.31.	7,496,623	5,541,966	1,890,187	48,710	15,760
1996.12.31.	7,829,353	5,677,631	2,085,568	50,514	15,640
1999.12.31.	16,261,889	5,238,149	10,822,302	32,868	168,570
2006.12.31.	17,739,939	8,604,823	9,086,368	26,991	21,757
2007.12.31.	18,266,742	9,149,209	9,063,143	27,242	27,148
2008.12.31.	18,335,409	9,493,444	8,781,483	27,614	32,868
2009.12.31.	18,623,845	9,866,681	8,679,861	36,368	40,935
2010.12.31.	19,228,875	10,414,780	8,674,492	90,222	49,381
2011.12.31.	19,885,911	10,976,501	8,675,430	171,134	62,846
2012.12.31.	20,329,060	11,464,198	8,568,396	207,890	88,576
2013.12.31.	20,744,780	11,935,759	8,514,434	177,569	117,018
2014.12.31.	21,125,135	12,309,856	8,444,710	202,536	168,033
2015.12.31.	21,568,354	12,805,852	8,302,809	240,582	219,111
2016.12.31.	21,832,524	13,192,436	8,060,199	296,757	283,132
2017.12.31.	21,824,172	13,459,240	7,691,917	327,723	345,292
2018.12.31.	22,313,869	13,817,963	7,694,885	330,422	470,599
2019.12.31.	22,216,229	14,157,574	7,232,063	328,727	497,865
2020.12.31.	22,107,028	14,320,025	6,898,118	362,328	526,557
2021.12.31.	22,347,586	14,580,825	6,827,009	396,632	543,120
2022.12.31.	22,497,819	14,785,761	6,845,744	365,487	500,827
2023. 1.31.	22,322,473	14,693,894	6,771,067	361,266	496,246

Source: National Pension Service National Pension Research Institute (2023: 1)

the total older adults. After the enactment of the National Pension Act in 1986, the national pension system actually started in 1988. The number of insured persons to the national pension increased fivefold from 4,433,695 as of the end of 1988 to 22,322,473 as of January 2023 [National Pension Service National Pension Research Institute, 2023](Table 5-1).

Changes in Social Welfare Services for Older Adults

Introduction of long-term care insurance system and expansion of national dementia management system

In most Western welfare countries, long-term care benefits for older adults are integrated into the health insurance system. On the other hand, along with Germany and Japan, Korea has established itself as an independent social insurance system. In other words, it is an independent long-term care insurance system for older adults, not an integrated one. On September 5, 1988, Korea announced the beginning of long-term care benefits by enacting ‘Regulations on the Establishment and Management of Nursing Facilities for Older Adults’, and in September 1995, Seoul Junggye Welfare Center for Older adults opened as the first nursing facility specializing in dementia [Ministry of Health and Welfare, 2001].

You can understand the history of long-term care benefits focusing on the national management of dementia. Since 1997, the operation of the Dementia Counseling and Reporting Center has begun. The center is responsible for registering and managing seniors with dementia, providing counseling and support for seniors with dementia and their caregivers, conducting education on the prevention of dementia and care tips for seniors with dementia, providing services to seniors at home with dementia as a guide for visits and management, and guiding admission to specialized nursing facilities for seniors with dementia [Ministry of Health and Welfare, 2001]. Since ‘Establishment of a Comprehensive Management and Support System for Older Adults with Dementia' was proposed in 'The First Basic Plan for Low Fertility and Aging Society' in September 2008, to manage comprehensive and systematic measures, 'The First National Dementia Plan (2008-2012)', 'The Second (2013-2016)', 'The Third (2017-2020)', and 'The Fourth (2021-2025)' have been established [Ministry of Health and Welfare, 2023]. Currently, the national accountability system for dementia is being implemented.

Expansion of welfare services at home for community integration

Following the trend of deinstitutionalization that began in the mid-1980s, it can be evaluated that home-based services have expanded with the introduction of the long-term care insurance system for older adults. Various forms of welfare services such as home nursing service from 1991, daycare service and short-term care service from 1992, began for older adults at home [Ministry of Health and Welfare, 2023]. As of 2001, welfare service for older adults at home was divided into a government support project for seniors aged 65 or older who are eligible for national basic livelihood security (free of charge) and targeting low-income seniors aged 65 or older (actual expenses), provided by the national govern- ments, local governments, social welfare corporations, and non-profit corporations [Ministry of Health and Welfare, 2001]. The number of commuting-system welfare facilities for senior citizens at home also increased continuously through the regulations on welfare services at the home of the 「Long-Term Care Insurance Act」 in 2007(Table 5-2). However, according to the direction of community integration service, short-term care service agencies decreased slightly.

Table 5-2. Changes in commuting-system welfare facilities for senior citizens at home : 2006-2021

(unit: number)

	2006	2007	2008	2009	2010	2011	2012	2013	2014	2015	2016	2017	2018	2019	2020	2021
total	1,045	1,408	2,298	2,696	2,496	2,750	3,003	2,832	2,797	3,089	3,168	3,216	3,494	4,821	7,212	9,984
home care service	523	767	1,111	1,228	1,118	1,180	1,113	1,042	992	1,021	1,009	1,001	1,051	1,513	2,656	4,156
day and night care service	409	504	621	714	786	842	840	848	913	1,007	1,086	1,174	1,312	1,816	2,321	2,618
short-term care service	-	-	217	288	67	95	94	110	96	112	95	80	73	78	73	69
visiting bath service	-	-	349	466	525	633	633	603	588	617	588	609	650	942	1,596	2,415
visiting nursing service	113	137	-	-	-	-	-	-	-	-	-	10	21	60	95	158
welfare equipment support service			-	-	-	-	-	-	-	-	-	-	-	0	86	208
home-based support service	-	-	-	-	-	-	323	229	208	332	390	342	387	412	385	360

Source: E-Country Index (2023). Current status of welfare facilities for senior citizens: commuting-system welfare facilities for senior citizens at home. (extracted 28 May 2023)

Expansion of leisure activities and social participation support services for older adults

Support for leisure services for older adults has also been expanded. On June 17, 1996, by the pilot installation of five welfare towns for older adults, older adults in the region could use medical care and nursing care as well as additional services such as sports, arts, and culture were available in one place [Ministry of Health and Welfare, 2001]. On October 2, 1998, by holding the launching ceremony of 'The Community Service Counselors' at the Second Senior Citizens' Day, lots of attention was paid to the participation of older adults in volunteer work [Ministry of Health and Welfare,

Table 5-3. Changes in leisure welfare facilities for senior citizens: 2006-2021

(unit: number)

division	2006	2007	2008	2009	2010	2011	2012	2013	2014	2015	2016	2017	2018	2019	2020	2021
senior welfare center	183	211	228	237	259	281	300	319	344	347	350	364	385	391	398	357
senior citizen center	55,504	56,480	57,930	59,543	60,737	61,537	62,442	63,251	63,960	64,568	65,044	65,604	66,286	66,737	67,316	67,211

Source: E-Country Index (2023). Current status of welfare facilities for senior citizens: Leisure welfare for senior citizens. (extracted 28 May 2023)

2001]. Many leisure facilities were also steadily expanded through the redefinition of leisure welfare facilities for senior citizens in the 「Welfare of Senior Citizens Act」 in 2007 and the introduction of the 「Framework Act on the Promotion of Leisure of Citizens」 in 2015(Table 5-3).

Transition to a customized care service for older adults and response to elder abuse

The care service for older adults began in 1987 with the dispatch project of home service workers. Afterwards, a series of care services began, and they were the living support project for older adults living alone and a senior caregiver voucher project in 2007, home care services in 2008, the life manager dispatch project for older adults living alone in 2009, support service project for home-based older adults in 2010, the community integrated care project in 2019, and the customized care service for older adults in 2020 [Min *et al.*, 2021]. As elder abuse emerged as a serious social problem, the number of care and protection service institutions for abused seniors increased(Table 5-4).

Table 5-4. Changes in older adults care and protective service institutions: 2006-2021

(unit: number)

division	2008	2009	2010	2011	2012	2013	2014	2015	2016	2017	2018	2019	2020	2021
elder protection agencies	20	21	24	25	25	25	28	29	29	32	33	34	35	37
shelters for elder abuse victims	-	-	-	-	-	-	-	-	-	-	18	19	19	20

Source: E-Country Index (2023). Current status of welfare facilities for senior citizens: Institutions specializing in protection for older adults, job support institutions for older adults, and shelters exclusively for abused seniors. (extracted 28 May 2023)

Transformation from senior competency bank to senior job support organization

Institutions for supporting work activities in old-age have been expanded and developed, such as the Senior Competency Bank in 1981, the Senior Shared Workspace in 1986, the Senior Employment Center in 1997, the Human Resources Development Agency for senior citizens, an agency helping senior citizens land a job and job placement agency for senior citizens since 2000. [Ministry of Health and Welfare, 2001; Ministry of Health and Welfare, 2023](Table 5-5).

Table 5-5. Changes in dedicated elderly employment agencies: 2015-2021

(unit: number)

division	2015	2016	2017	2018	2019	2020	2021
dedicated elderly employment agencies	129	136	153	160	184	196	206

Source: E-Country Index (2023). Current status of welfare facilities for senior citizens: dedicated elderly employment agencies. (extracted 28 May 2023)

Summary

Over the past 60 years, Korean welfare for older adults has shown remarkable growth, expanding the comprehensiveness of the system, expanding the coverage, and increasing the level of benefits. However, problems such as poverty, the blind spot of care, and the gap in welfare between urban and rural areas for older adults are still exposed. In particular, policies at the national level for long-lived older adults are practically absent.

What should be the direction of social welfare policy for centenarians in Korea? In a word, the direction is the establishment of the 'Longevity Perspective'. Along with the entry into the intelligent information society, we are witnessing an increase in the number of long-lived and healthy people due to the quantum jump development of human science and medicine. The increase in the longevity population in this society is not an increase in risk and burden, but it is necessary to sublimate it to a productive approach of passing statecraft on the economy and a humanistic approach of awe of life. That approach can be the expansion of a longevity cognitive perspective in all areas of law and policy for long-lived seniors. As a concrete social welfare system, the income security policy for centenarians needs to be designed in terms of additional benefits. It is the so-called longevity allowance. Second, it is necessary to introduce customized longevity services for the super-aged. Longevity services for the super-aged need to be customized, such as nutrition service, home care caregiver system, companion service for lifetime reminiscence, treatment and leisure service for caregivers, and funeral service.

References

- E-Country Index. Current Status of Welfare Facilities for senior citizens. (https://www.index.go.kr/unity/potal/indicator/ProgressIndicator.do?cdNo=210) (retrieved on April 30, 2021). Daejeon : Statistics Korea, 2021.
- Lee HL. Dying of old age in Japan : what happens with the collapse of older adults care and care in 2025. Jeju National University Graduate School of Interpretation and Translation Master's thesis, 2018.
- Min SY *et al*. A study on how to activate cooperation in connection with local community public sector case management. Seoul : Social Security Information Service, Suwon : Kyonggi University Industry-University Cooperation Foundation, 2021.
- Ministry of Health and Welfare. 2001 Senior Health Welfare Government Subsidy Guidelines. Sejong : Ministry of Health and Welfare, 2001.
- Ministry of Health and Welfare. 2023 Older adults Health and Welfare Business Guide I. Sejong : Ministry of Health and Welfare, 2023a.
- Ministry of Health and Welfare. 2023 Older adults Health and Welfare Business Guide Ⅱ. Sejong : Ministry of Health and Welfare, 2023b.
- Ministry of Health and Welfare. 2023 Dementia Policy Business Guide. Sejong : Ministry of Health and Welfare, 2023c.
- National Pension Service National Pension Research Institute. National pension published statistics (as of the end of January 2023). (https://institute.nps.or.kr/jsppage/research/resources/resources_05.jsp) (retrieved on 28 May 2023). Jeonju : National Pension Service National Pension Research Institute, 2023.
- OECD. Pension at a Glance 2013: OECD and G20 Indicators. OECD iLibrary, 2013.

Chapter 06

Gerotranscendence of Korean Centenarians

Minjeong An

The aging of our country is progressing very rapidly due to the increase in life expectancy caused by advancements in medical technology and a decrease in the birth rate. According to the United Nations' population classification criteria [United Nations, 2019], South Korea entered an aging society with more than 7% of the population aged 65 and over in the year 2000, and it is becoming evident that we are entering a super-aged society with more than 20% of the population aged 65 and over in 2025, which is 25 years later [Statistics Korea, 2022]. This aging trend is not unique to South Korea but is also a global phenomenon, including the United Kingdom, Canada, and Poland expected to enter a super-aged society like South Korea in 2025 [Statistics Korea, 2022].

We are approaching longevity, which many consider a blessing. However, as it aligns with the declining birth rate, society is aging overall. Consequently, issues such as labor shortages, economic slowdown, and increased economic burdens due to the healthcare and support of the elderly have emerged, resulting in a generally negative perception of older people in society. This negative perception soon affects middle-aged and younger individuals who will quickly become elderly, deepening the problem further [Statistics Korea, 2021]. Therefore, as we stand on the brink of entering a super-aged society, it is essential to urgently change these negative perceptions towards older people and foster a correct understanding of the aging process.

Alongside these negative views of older people, several concepts have emerged, focusing on positive perspectives such as active aging, successful aging, well-aging, and smart aging. In academia, there is particular attention to the concept of "gerotranscendence," introduced by Swedish gerontologist Tornstam in 1994, within the framework of positive aging theory [Tornstam L, 1996]. Notable psychologists like Erikson, known for his stages of psychosocial development, originally proposed eight stages of development for individuals over the age of 60, culminating in ego integrity or despair. However, in light of increasing life expectancy and the realization that the psychosocial stages for individuals over the age of 60 may not be the same for the next 20-30 years, up to 80-90 years or beyond, criticism emerged. Consequently, they incorporated the concept of gerotranscendence into the existing eight stages and completed the model by expanding human psychosocial development into a total of nine stages [Erikson EH and Erikson JM, 1998].

Gerotranscendence is a compound word in English derived from the ancient Greek "gero," meaning old age, and Latin "transcendence," signifying going beyond and it represents a concept that pursues a fulfilling life in mature old age [Tornstam L, 2005]. Gerotranscendence occurs as the elderly transition from a materialistic and rational worldview to a more cosmic and transcendental one. As individuals age, they undergo continuous aging processes and encounter various crises and challenges in life that they may not have experienced before. How they perceive and cope with these challenges determines whether they break free from the limitations they once had and move forward into a new phase of life, reshaping the value of their existence. At this juncture, gerotranscendence is believed to be significantly related to the life satisfaction of the elderly, making it a noteworthy predictor for enhancing their life satisfaction.

Gerotranscendence is said to manifest in three dimensions: the cosmic dimension, the dimension of the self, and the dimension of social and personal relationships [Tornstam L, 2011]. In his work, Tornstam further elaborated on the three dimensions of gerotranscendence to help understand the changes that occur within each dimension. In the cosmic dimension, he identified five specific areas where the gerotranscendence change begins: time and childhood, the connection to earlier generations, life and death, mystery in life, and transcendental sources of happiness. These areas signify the beginning of a change in older people's perception of the cosmos [Tornstam L, 2005].

In the dimension of the self, he identified five specific areas where changes can be observed: self-confrontation, decrease in self-enteredness, development of body-transcendence, self-transcendence, and ego-integrity. These areas provide signals for changes in the self-perception of the elderly. In the dimension of social and personal relationships, Tornstam highlighted several areas where changes occur: changed meaning and importance of relations, role play, emancipated innocence, modern asceticism, and transcendence towards everyday wisdom. These areas reflect the evolving dynamics in older people's social and interpersonal relationships as they age and experience gerotranscendence [Tornstam L, 2005].

It's indeed fascinating to explore how gerotranscendence manifests in elderly individuals, particularly centenarians, in South Korea. Similar phenomena have been observed in neighboring countries like Japan, where some elderly individuals have exhibited gerotranscendence [Tomizawa K, 2009; Masui Y *et al.*, 2018]. In Taiwan, there have been reports suggesting a connection between gerotranscendence, life satisfaction, and religion among the elderly [Hsieh L-Y and Wang J-J, 2008; Liu K and Chen JM, 2022].

Understanding how gerotranscendence is expressed in centenarians and other elderly individuals in South Korea is an intriguing area of study. Centenarians born in 1917, as of the year 2022, have lived through significant historical events such as the Japanese colonial period and the Korean War, experiencing the transition before and after the establishment of the Republic of Korea. They grew up during a time when the social systems, including welfare, were being formed and stabilized. Many of them assumed the responsibility of caring for their families during their middle-aged years, but as they aged, they often did not receive the same level of support in return. This unique life experience, coupled with the physical aspect of living to be over a hundred years old, raises questions about what kind of psychosocial development these centenarians may have undergone in their later years.

Research into the psychological and social development of South Korea's centenarians can provide valuable insights into their experiences, perspectives, and the factors contributing to their well-being in old age. It can shed light on how their life experiences have shaped their perceptions of aging and how they have navigated the challenges and opportunities that come with extreme old age.

To conduct this study, we focused on 16 centenarians aged 95 and above residing in Jeollanam-do, South Korea, specifically in Gurye, Gokseong, Suncheon, and Damyang. From July to August 2022, we conducted surveys to gather demographic characteristics, disease-related information, and subjective well-being. Additionally, we conducted in-depth interviews applying a phenomenological method to explore their experiences in later life for those aged 65 and older.

Participant selection criteria included the ability to read, hear, understand, and respond to the survey questions in Korean. Exclusion criteria applied to individuals diagnosed with dementia or any psychiatric diseases. Jeollanam-do, with a senior population representing 25.2% of the total population as of 2022, is already advancing towards a super-aged society [Statistics Korea, 2023]. This region is also renowned for its high life expectancy, with an average life expectancy of 83-84 years (male: 79-80 years, female: 87-88 years) in 2020, making it a representative region for longevity in South Korea.

Our research team consisted of five members who received training in qualitative research methods. Efforts were made to standardize the interview process through training and pilot interviews. During the interviews, participants were asked about their life experiences since becoming elderly, and, when necessary, hearing aids were provided to facilitate communication. The interview data were analyzed independently by each team member, and categorized into three main domains and their sub-domains, following Tornstam's (2005) model for the development of gerotranscendence.

Therefore, this study aimed to gain insights into the experiences and characteristics of centenarians in South Korea, specifically those residing in regions with severe aging and a reputation for longevity.

Table 6-1. General characteristics of the study participants (N=16)

Characteristics		n	(%)	Mean±SD	Range
Age				97.31±1.45	95~100
Sex	Male	4	25.0		
	Female	12	75.0		
Education (year)				1.14±0.36	1~2
	1	12	75.0		
	2	2	12.5		
	Missing	2	12.5		
Cohabitat	Yes	3	18.8		
	No	9	56.3		
	Missing	4	25.0		
Residential area	Gurye	2	39.1		
	Gokseong	9	8.7		
	Damyang	4	17.4		
	Sunchang	1	4.3		
Number of children				6.20±1.21	4~8
	〈6	5	31.3		
	≥6	10	62.5		
	Missing	1	6.3		
Hypertension	Yes	8	50.0		
Diabetes	Yes	1	6.3		
Cardiovascular dz	Yes	1	6.3		
Arthritis	Yes	3	18.8		
Cancer	Yes	-			
	Yes	-			
Osteoporosis	Yes	-			
Smoking status	Yes	3	18.8		
Drinking status	Yes	15	72.2		
Sleeping (hour)				7.90±1.37	6~10
Infection of COVID-19	Yes	3	18.8		

Characteristics	n	(%)	Mean±SD	Range
Perceived happiness			3.69±0.85	2~5
1	-	-		
2	1	6.3		
3	4	25.0		
4	6	37.5		
5	2	12.5		
Missing	3	18.8		

The research included surveys, face-to-face in-depth interviews, and rigorous data analysis to explore the concept of gerotranscendence in this unique demographics.

Firstly, here are the general characteristics of the centenarians who participated in the interviews(Table 6-1). The average age was 97.3 years (ranging from 95 to 100). The majority were female, comprising 75.0% (n=12) of the participants. Their average educational duration was 1.14 ± 0.36 years, and all of them had been married at some point in their lives. These centenarians had been residing in the same homes since their marriage or since they became elderly.

As for their living situations, 56.3% (n=9) lived alone, while 18.8% (n=3) lived with others, and 25.0% (n=4) did not respond to this question. On average, they had 6.20 ± 1.21 children, with an average of 3.10 sons and 3.92 daughters. The majority of participants resided in Gokseong-gun, accounting for 39.1% (n=9) of the sample. Other participants were from Damyang-gun (4), Gurye-gun (2), and Suncheon-gun (1).

Concerning care services, 37.5% (n=6) of the participants were receiving long-term care services. The frequency of services varied based on care ratings and economic circumstances, ranging from 3 to 7 visits per week. These services included meal delivery, medication delivery, cleaning, errand running, and home bathing services, provided by caregivers based on individual needs.

The health conditions reported by these individuals were as follows: 8 individuals (50.0%) had high blood pressure (hypertension), 3 individuals (19.0%) had arthritis (joint inflammation), 1 individual (6.3%) had diabetes, and 1 individual (6.3%) had heart disease. There were no reported cases of cancer, kidney disease, osteoporosis, or other such illnesses. Three individuals (18.8%) reported being smokers, while another three individuals (18.8%) reported consuming alcohol. The average sleep duration was 7.90 ± 1.37 hours. Regarding COVID-19, three individuals (18.8%) reported having been infected with the virus but had since recovered.

To assess their subjective well-being, participants were asked to rate their current happiness on a 5-point Likert scale (1 = not happy at all, 5 = extremely happy). The average score was 3.69 ± 0.85 points, with 12 individuals (75.0%) reporting a moderate level of happiness or higher.

The First Stage of Gerotranscendence: Cosmic Dimension

In this stage, elderly individuals experience a sense of unity with the universe. They undergo a reevaluation of time, space, and objects, perceiving life and death differently from before. The fear of death diminishes, and there is an increased sense of intimacy between past and future generations. Tornstam identifies specific sub-domains within this stage: (1) Time and Childhood: This involves a shift in the perception of time, where the distinction between today and yesterday blurs, allowing for the coexistence of different time periods; (2) The Connection to Earlier Generations: This sub-omain encompasses a growing sense of being part of the flow of earlier generations; (3) Life and Death: Individuals experience a change in their perception of life and death, resulting in reduced death anxiety; (4) Mystery in Life: This involves accepting aspects of life that cannot be explained by science or reason; and (5) Transcendental Sources of Happiness: Happiness expands from grand experiences to subtle, everyday moments, allowing individuals to experience the vastness of the universe through the small cosmos of their lives.

Based on our interviews results, changes in the perception of life and death, corresponding to the third sub-domain, were validated in six female centenarians. They exhibited a more comfortable and familiar acceptance of death, as elaborated below.

(Case 1) She is a 99-year-old female and got married at the age of sixteen and lived with her husband until he passed away at the age of 65. Currently, at the age of 99, she lives alone. She had two sons and four daughters, but she expressed sadness because two of her daughters passed away before her. Recently, her son remodeled the house, and she was delighted that the outdoor bathroom was moved inside. She also noticed that safety bars were installed in the living room, which doubles as the kitchen, to assist her with walking.

"I've lived well up to now (since I've lived), and it's time for me to go (because I've lived). I'm worried about going (dying). I'm worried about dying. I want to go peacefully, as if I'm going to sleep. I don't

have any other worries. I go to church and sit quietly in a chair, and it would be nice if I died there. I'm praying for that now. Don't let me live until I'm a hundred; just take me when it's time, God. ··· I don't have any other worries at all (smiles). I'm not afraid of death because when I die, I'll go to heaven"

(Case 2) She is a 95-year-old female and got married at the age of seventeen and had one son and one daughter. After her husband passed away, she lived alone for 72 years, working on her farm. Her son and daughter-in-law retired and moved to her hometown, living nearby. She mentioned that she had lived relatively comfortably throughout her life and had never faced financial difficulties.

"When it's time to die, I should just die. But I haven't died yet. I think, 'I'm this old now; why am I not dying?'··· These thoughts come to me, alone. It's nice to live. Living is nice, but now that I'm supposed to die, why am I not dying? What am I going to do··· Thoughts like that come to me. I've gotten really old now···"

(Case 3) The woman is 98 years old and got married at the age of 20. She had four sons and five daughters, all of whom are still alive. She currently lives with her daughter. She proudly displays a photo on her wall that includes more than 30 descendants, including children and grandchildren. She recalls the photo was taken when her daughters wore traditional Korean clothing (hanbok) and her sons wore ties, and she describes it as a very happy time. As her mobility decreased, she enjoys sitting by the open door, watching cars pass by on the distant road, observing the sunrise and sunset, and appreciating the blooming and withering of flowers.

"Now that my body has become cumbersome, it's better to just

pass away; that's the best. My body is just heavy now. Dying would be comfortable. It's good to do nothing. The other world is good, so once you go there (as a deceased person), you don't come back."

Next, there was a centenarian who experienced the mystery of life corresponding to the fourth subcategory. In the past, he thought he was firmly grounded in the world. However, recently, he has been having mystical experiences, seeing themselves floating in the universe in dreams or during meditation. He usually reads the Bible and engages in meditation frequently these days.

(Case) A 97-year-old man, who used to be a pastor for over a decade, had been in good health until last year when he could still walk well. However, starting from this spring, his legs began to swell, and his health deteriorated. He has six daughters, and the third daughter visits him frequently and talks to him. He usually spends his time reading the Bible and meditating, with Korean and world maps on the wall, praying and meditating.

*"I read the Bible and meditate a lot. For example, simple yet difficult questions··· Why does life exist··· Who am I··· What I feel these days is that the universe is infinitely vast. It's endless. There's no end to it. I feel like we are floating in the universe··· There's nothing to envy··· Even death (is not scary)··· I feel that God has sh*own mercy to me, so I don't feel fear, and I can go before God···"

In addition to the responses related to the fifth sub-domain of the first area, which is "transcendental sources of happiness," the main responses to the interview questions were not directly related to this sub-domain. However, expressions of gratitude and joy in everyday life experiences that help oneself were observed.

"I don't have anything more to wish for, and I don't want to wish for more by pushing it. I live as I'm given. I don't want to live longer, and I don't want to die either. I leave it to fate. It's unavoidable. No matter how good things are, I might not know they're good, and even if I see bad things, I might not know they're bad. The world is just the way it is. I've lived like this and found it enjoyable… Even if I live like this, if I don't die, what can I do? (…ellipsis…) Nowadays, the staff from the local office come and ask me why I'm thinking about repaying the debt… I'm grateful… Because of that… I'm thankful, so they come to bathe me again today and wash me, and they're so happy… Why would they do so much for someone like me …(Female, 95 years old)."

These are the sentiments expressed by Kim, a 102-year-old woman, reflecting on her life and the happiness she found in her relationship with her husband and the company of friends.

"I was always happy while living with my husband. We had a good relationship. So, those times were happy. It was always good. He used to say that we didn't need to worry about things outside, as long as we raised our children well. It was good back then. I have no regrets… My heart is always happy. I never feel lonely. I watch television and hang out with friends so I don't feel lonely. Because I always live with a good heart, it feels like I've lived a long life. It's always been good. There has never been a bad time. (Female, 102 years old)."

"Now, I live comfortably. I cook my own meals, just go out to gatherings, then come home and sleep… When my children call, I

answer, my son-in-law in Gwangju calls, and my sons call in the evening··· It's cold, but stay warm and sleep··· (My children) call me thinking about me, so they call···(Female, 96 years old)."

PART II

The Second Stage of Transcending old age: The Dimension of the Self

In this stage, elderly individuals discover the hidden aspects of their self, including both the positive and negative sides. They redefine their self-concept, experience a reduced interest in material possessions, and move away from placing themselves at the center of the universe. Instead, they focus on self-care without obsessing over their health, experience moments of regression to their childhood, and gain insights that life's puzzle pieces form a complete whole.

Tornstam identifies the following sub-dimensions within this stage: (1) Self-confrontation: The process of discovering one's hidden facets, including strengths and weaknesses; (2) Decrease in self-centeredness: Shifting away from viewing oneself as the center of the universe; (3) Development of body-transcendence: Continuing to care for one's body without becoming overly fixated on it; (4) Self-transcendence: Transitioning from a self-centered focus to greater concern for others, particularly children and grandchildren (more common in males); (5) Ego-integrity: Realizing that individual life puzzle pieces contribute to the formation of the complete puzzle, signifying a delicate state requiring both serenity and solitude.

The interview results from this study with centenarians showed that the sub-dimension of body-transcendence was prominently observed. Additionally, elements of self-confrontation, transitioning from individualism to altruism (self-transcendence), and a sense of maintaining serenity were identified in these elderly participants as part of their self-transcendence in old age.

(Case 1) This 95-year-old woman remarried to a man from a southern province and had a daughter when she was 42. Her daughter now lives nearby and brings her food twice a day, taking care of her meals. She feels grateful and happy for her daughter's help and the way her daughter looks after her.

"This is how my fate has been from the beginning… I don't know what it's like to feel lonely or anything like that. I think it's time to go because I've lived long enough. Is there any point in living too long? I read books. But now, my age has caught up with me, and my eyes have gotten worse. I wish my eyes hadn't deteriorated like this. But even now, my eyes are better than they should be for my age. It's tough to see, but I read books. Even though it's hard to see, that's my joy in life."

(Case 2) This 97-year-old woman got married at 20 into a family with 18 members, including 10 sisters-in-law. She had a challenging life adapting to her large family but lived a good life until her husband passed away five years ago. She feels thankful for her daughters, who now take care of her, but she also has a sense of regret that her daughters have to work hard because of her.

"My hearing isn't as good as it used to be. I could hear things slightly back then, but now, if someone speaks softly, I can't hear them well. But it's okay if I can't hear. I don't mind not hearing. So, even if I don't hear it properly, I just let it be… (trails off). I had

a broken spine. They wouldn't perform surgery on me. They said I was too weak for it. They refused to do the surgery, saying I might not wake up if they did it. I went to Gwangju and Suncheon, but they wouldn't operate. So now, I'm trying to walk and endure it··· I just manage as it is··· When I'm in too much pain, I go for a painkiller injection and come back. After that, when I feel better, I go somewhere. Maybe I'll go to the market or somewhere else. It's been about 20 years like this. But even though I live like this without my husband, I have no complaints. It's all good."

(Case 3) This 98-year-old man lives with his second wife, who is currently 83 years old, after his first wife passed away. He has 3 sons and 5 daughters. He faced economic hardships throughout his life but finds happiness in his children, who occasionally contact him and visit. He expresses a sense of loneliness as there are no other elderly men of his age around. Recently, the joy of having great-grandchildren is a significant source of happiness for him.

"Spinal stenosis makes walking uncomfortable, but I endure it and walk around the neighborhood every day. There are no men my age around, so it's boring. Though my body isn't as active, it's not necessarily good to live a long life··· I should consider that I've lived this long because I took care of my health. I didn't drink or smoke, so my stomach should be in good condition. I didn't have a selective diet; I ate various foods. I should say that I've lived a long life because I took care of my health."

(Case 4) *"I was born during the Japanese colonial period, and when I was 25, the Korean War broke out. At that time, they drafted all the young people into the People's Army. I went into hiding because I had gotten married. I wondered why I was even born. Why was I born··· I searched for God for ten years··· Looking back, even that* *was God's plan. So, what we think is unfortunate may have some happiness, and what we feel is happiness may also be unfortunate. We humans think we're unhappy, but in reality, other creatures are using humans. In the end, humans aren't the ones who are unhappy. I came to realize that."*

The Third Stage of Transcending old age: The Dimension of Social and Personal Relationships

In this stage, the elderly reduce unnecessary relationships, decrease materialistic desires, and become more interested in inner activities. Tornstam identifies specific areas within this dimension: (1) Changed Meaning and Importance of Relations: Individuals make choices about superficial relationships, and their interest in such relationships diminishes. They gradually feel the need for solitude, signifying a change in the significance of relationships; (2) Role Play: People understand the differences between themselves and the roles they've played throughout life. Sometimes, they let go of these roles and transcend them to get closer to their true selves; (3) Emancipated Innocence: This involves surpassing unnecessary societal norms, conventions, and rules, gaining new abilities that allow individuals to break free from these constraints; (4) Modern Asceticism: It signifies the shift away from efforts to fulfill materialistic needs and desires that were important in the past. Instead, individuals begin to give to their children, grandchildren, and others. (5) Everyday Wisdom: This aspect involves transcending the duality of right and wrong, withholding judgment, and discerning advice. It accompanies an open heart and tolerance. These elements collectively describe the third stage of transcending old age.

The interview results of this study revealed that the dimension of everyday wisdom was typically apparent in the transcendence of the social and personal relationship dimension among centenarians. They belonged to a generation deeply rooted in Confucian culture, where respecting and visiting one's parents was considered a matter of course. However, they displayed a transcendent attitude toward their busy children.

A 100-year-old woman, born in her hometown, got married at 18, had five children, and had never left her hometown. She still enjoyed working in her vegetable garden and felt both gratitude and guilt about her youngest son visiting her about once a week.

> *"At this point, there's nothing that's particularly good or bad. There's nothing to regret, nothing special. I'm getting older, and even if it gets cold, it's okay. Even if my children don't come to see me, as long as they manage their households and raise their own families well. They all got married, so they could raise their children and manage their households. Whether they come to see me or not, it doesn't matter. I trust them, and even if they always come and go, there's no problem. Just live well without any issues. It's better to keep living like this and go when it's time."*

Another 96-year-old woman, who originally lived in Seoul, moved to the countryside at the age of 15, got married, and worked as a farmer. After her husband passed away at age 40, she struggled to raise her three daughters independently. Now, she lives alone, but her daughters visit and take care of her.

"My father had a lot of money, and a close friend from the Independence Movement asked him for some money a couple of times. He helped him, but when the Japanese army found out, they started investigating my father, so we had to flee to the countryside. My father passed away three years later. Since then, life was a constant struggle. I raised my children like silkworms··· Now, all my children are grown up and married··· Now I can live comfortably. I lie down, sit up, watch TV, and when I'm quiet, I think of my deceased children, my living children, the things I used to do in the past··· Even thoughts from before I got married and thoughts about my parents and siblings··· I still think about them. Even after getting married, I still think about them··· I just hope my children stay healthy and live well. That's what I think about."

Summary

Our research results indicate that centenarians have reached some stages of transcending aging in three dimensions: the cosmic dimension, the dimension of the self, and the dimension of social and personal relationships. Additionally, the subjective happiness of the participants was rated at an average of 3.69 points on a 5-point scale, indicating moderate happiness. Transcending aging can develop or progress differently based on cultural and life experiences and is not experienced by all elderly individuals. However, studies suggest that those who undergo transcending aging experience lower levels of anxiety and depression and increased life satisfaction.

Our study participants, being individuals who have experienced significant historical events (i.e., Independence war, civil war), in their lives, raised concerns that deep-seated sadness and anxiety might inhibit or interfere with the process of transcending aging. However, we found evidence of varying levels of transcending aging in our participants. This could be attributed to the influence of our culture, which has been shaped by Eastern philosophies such as Confucianism and Buddhism, where the concept of transcendence may be inherent to some extent. Furthermore, our participants were predominantly healthy centenarians who, while exhibiting some degree of frailty, still maintained a certain level of independent functioning, a factor that could have influenced these findings.

Many of the previous gerotranscendence studies in our country focused on seniors aged 60 and above. However, our research holds significance as it analyzed face-to-face interviews with centenarians to confirm gerotranscendence. While there have been studies abroad investigating gerotranscendence in various age groups of elderly individuals, it was challenging to find research that specifically explored the basis of gerotranscendence in those aged 95 and older.

In this regard, our research findings can contribute to a deeper understanding of centenarians' gerotranscendence both domestically and internationally. They can serve as foundational data for the development of policies and programs aimed at guiding older people toward gerotranscendence. Ultimately, this can enhance the positive perception of aging and contribute to the increased life satisfaction and well-being of centenarians. Since our research was based on qualitative analysis of interviews with centenarians, future studies should utilize gerotranscendence scales to assess the extent of gerotranscendence among centenarians in our country quantitatively. Additionally, research to examine the relationships between gerotranscendence and psychological and social variables such as depression, anxiety, and life satisfaction is needed.

References

- Erikson EH, Erikson JM. The life cycle completed (extended version). New York (NY): WW Norton & Company, 1998.
- Hsieh L-Y, Wang J-J. The relationship between gerotranscendence and demographics in institutionalized elders. Journal of Nursing. 2008;55(6): 37-46.
- Liu K, Chen JM. The mindset, lifelong learning, and gerotranscendence of elderly women in Taiwan: An exploratory study. Women's Studies International Forum. 2022;90:102552.
- Masui Y, Gondo Y, Yasumoto S, *et al.* Caregiving experience promotes the growth of gerotranscendence in old age. Innovation in Aging. 2018; 2(Suppl 1):290.
- Statistics Korea [Internet]. 2022 older people statistics. Dae Jeon (Republic of Korea); c2022 [cited 2023 Sep 22]. Available from: https://kostat.go.kr/synap/skin/doc.html?fn=44fc580646bd977f4b72b1e4523aeb799f43db0045f93b133958e4cb6ca69ae6&rs=/synap/preview/board/10820/
- Statistics Korea [Internet]. Future population projections. Dae Jeon (Republic of Korea); c2021 [cited 2023 Sep 22]. Available from: https://kosis.kr/statHtml/statHtml.do?orgId=101&tblId=DT_1BPA004&conn_path=I2
- Statistics Korea [Internet]. Proportion of elderly population. Dae Jeon (Republic of Korea); c2023 [cited 2023 Sep 22]. Available from: https://kosis.kr/statHtml/statHtml.do?orgId=101&tblId=DT_1YL20631&conn_path=I2.
- Tomizawa K. Gerotranscendence in everyday life among the oldest old in the amama achipelago. Japanese Journal of Gerontology. 2009;30(4):477-488.
- Tornstam L. Caring for the elderly: introducing the theory of gerotranscendence as a supplementary frame of reference for caring for the elderly. Scandinavian Journal of Caring Sciences. 1996;10(3):144-150.
- Tornstam L. Gerotranscendence: a developmental theory of positive aging. New York (NY): Springer Publishing Company Inc.; 2005.

- Tornstam L. Maturing into gerotranscendence. Journal of Transpersonal Psychology. 2011;43(2):166-180.
- United Nations Department of Economic and Social Affairs [Internet]. World Population Prospects 2019: Methodology of the United Nations population estimates and projections. New York (NY); c2019 [cited 2023 Sep 23]. Available from: https://population.un.org/wpp/Publications/Files/WPP2019_Methodology.pdf

PART III

CHANGES IN HEALTH STATUS AND LIFESTYLE OF KOREAN CENTENARIANS

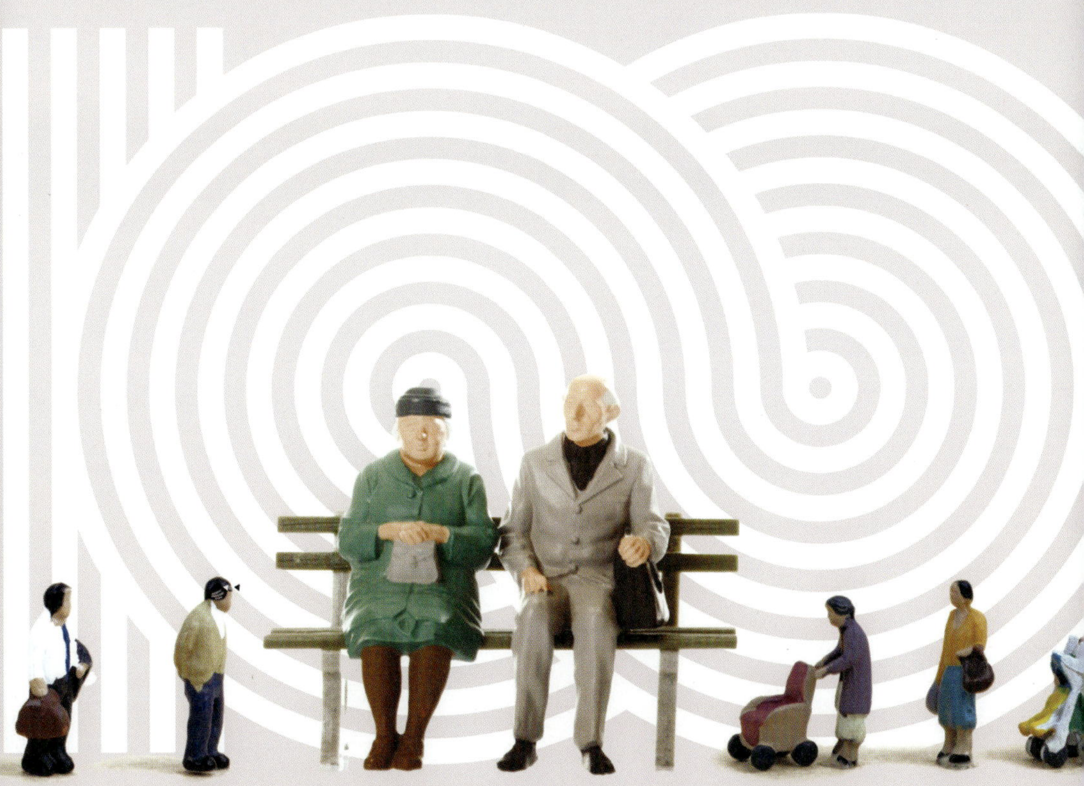

Chapter 07

Physical and Mental Health Status of Korean Centenarians

Kwangsung Park and Min Jhon

Introduction

Data from the National Statistical Office indicates a remarkable increase in the number of centenarians in Korea, from approximately 900 in the early 2000s to 4,819 in 2019, translating to 9.6 per 100,000 population. The number of centenarians gradually increased, following 459 in 1990, 494 in 1995, 1,835 in 2010, and 3,159 in 2015. Notably, while the proportion of female centenarians remains high, the male percentage has gradually increased — from 10.8% in 2005 to 15.2% in 2020(Figure 7-1).

Exceptional longevity is mainly influenced by genetic, lifestyle, and environmental factors [Evert J, 2003, Govindaraju D, 2015]. It was suggested that longevity could be affected by interaction among variables such as genes, sex, habitat, nutrition, physical activity, social care, and lifestyle [Park SC, 2012].

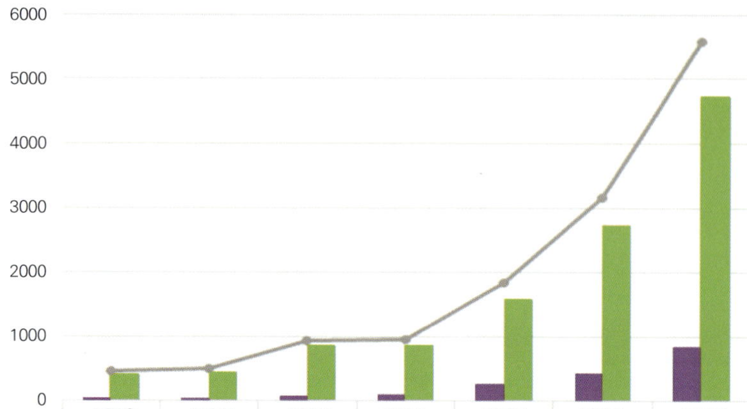

	1990	1995	2000	2005	2010	2015	2020
men	45	42	82	104	255	428	850
women	414	452	852	856	1,580	2,731	4,731
total	459	494	934	960	1,835	3,159	5,581

Figure 7-1. The centenarians in Korea from 2000 to 2020. This data is adapted from the Korean statistical information service.

In 2001, the Korean centenarian team led by professor Sang Chul Park conducted a nationwide Korean centenarians study. They selected 11 counties in Korea based on a super longevity index and a longevity index reported by the Korean National Statistical Office [Park SC, 2008]. After the nationwide Korean centenarian study, the southwestern area of the Korean peninsula, specifically 4 counties (Gurye gun, Goksong gun, Sunchang gun, and Damyang gun, abbreviated as the GuGokSunDam area), was designated as the representative long-life zone in Korea [Park SC, 2012].

In 2018, the Korean Centenarians Study Group undertook a comprehensive study in the GuGokSunDam region(Figure 7-2), with the findings subsequently published in 2021 [Park K *et. al.*, 2021]. This chapter provides an in-depth review of the shifts in the mental

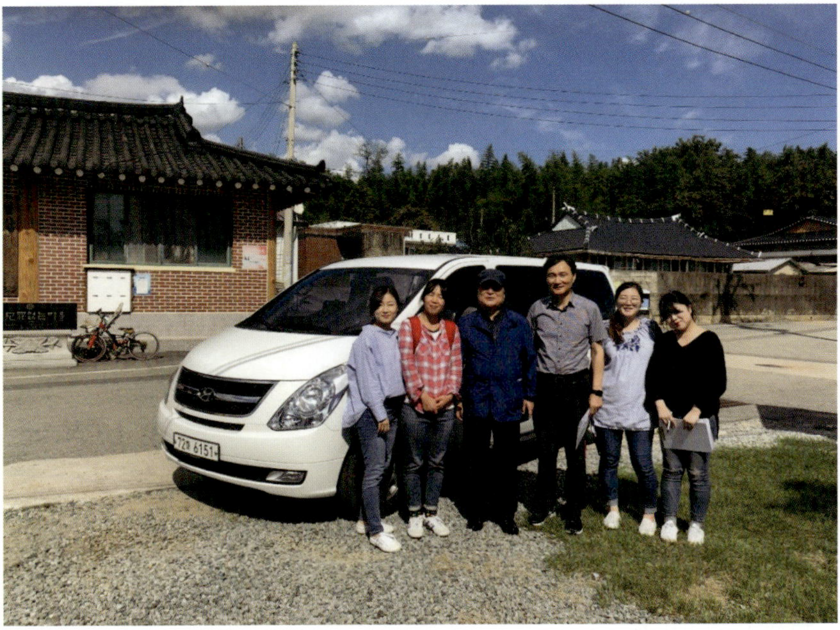

Figure 7-2. **Members of the 2018 Korea centenarian study group during the field study.** At the center are Professor Sang Chul Park and Kwangsung Park

and physical well-being of Korean centenarians over 20 years, drawing extensively from the referenced work [Park K *et. al.*, 2021].

Changes in the Physical and Mental Health of Korean Centenarians in 20 years

In 2001, 72 subjects (5 male and 67 female) in the GuGokSunDam area participated in the Korean centenarian study. The age range of centenarians was 100-112, and the mean age was 102.3. The ratio of males to females was 1:13, and the overall health status of males tended to be good compared to women. In 2018, a total of

37 centenarians (6 male, 31 female) in the same area participated in the survey, with an average age of 101.8 and an age range of 100-107 years. The male-to-female ratio was 1:5, indicating the male population increase in 2018. In developed countries such as the United States, the male-to-female ratio of centenarians was reported to be about 1:4-5, indicating that the ratio of GuGokSunDam centenarians in 2018 is changing to the developed type compared to 2001.

Lifestyle and physical health status of centenarians

The subjective health status of centenarians is generally reported to be good. It showed 65.3% of good to very good in 2001, and 63.7% in 2018. However, subjective health status does not reflect objective health status because subjective health status reflects physical and mental health status and socioeconomic status [Araújo L *et al.*, 2018].

Lifestyle factors, including smoking and alcohol consumption, are widely acknowledged as health risks that diminish the quality of life [Ng R *et al.*, 2020]. Smoking has been identified to reduce life expectancy [Cicconetti P, 2002]. In the study of 2018, 75.0% of centenarians did not smoke during their lifetime, and the ratio of lifetime non-smokers was higher than the 2001 survey result (60.0%). With regard to alcohol consumption, the 2001 survey indicated that 20.0% of centenarians consumed alcohol, whereas by 2018, 6.1% of centenarians reported current alcohol consumption. Centenarians reported an average sleep duration of 9.0 hours. When comparing those who slept for more than 9 hours, the percentage dropped from 72.5% in 2001 to 53.8% in 2018.

In the laboratory findings of the Korean centenarian study in

2001, there were no significant differences between men and women in the laboratory findings except in diastolic blood pressure and serum creatinine levels. The mean blood pressure was higher in women (149.3/86.6mmHg) compared to men (136.3/76.4mmHg). The total cholesterol level was similar in both men (174.6± 29.6mg/dl) and women (174.6±37.2mg/dl), which is relatively lower than those in the general old people. The mean serum glucose level was 115.9 in men and 104.3 mg/dl in women. The reason for higher glucose levels in men was 2 cases of diabetes. The average BMI was 21.9kg/m^3 in men and 20.9kg/m^3 in women.

In old age, physical functions deteriorate due to frailty or cognitive impairment, making it difficult to carry out daily life alone, and sometimes people need help from people around them. The ability to perform daily living is a tool to evaluate whether older adults can live independently and is widely used to evaluate the level of functioning in older adults.

In the centenarians' survey in 2001, looking at the ability to perform daily activities, 77.9% of people could use the bathroom alone, eat 73.6%, change clothes 72.3%, move 63.9%, and take a bath 45.8%. In 2018, 82.9% of the participants ate alone, 65.7% used the bathroom, 57.1% were moving, 43.9% were changing clothes, and 22.9% bathed.

A distinction emerges from the basic daily living performance skills in assessing instrumental activities of daily living (IADLs) necessary for social life. In 2018, centenarians, relative to their 2001 counterparts, were more self-sufficient across all evaluated areas, irrespective of living arrangements. Notably, elderly individuals residing alone demonstrated greater independence in all areas than those living with family or in care facilities. Nevertheless, among centenarians living alone, there remains a pronounced dependency: 66.7% required assistance with tasks such as shopping, using transportation (66.7%), performing household chores (44.4%), and making telephone calls (11.1%). These findings underscore the pressing need for local government and public sectors to bolster support services. The detailed daily living performance skills of centenarians will be discussed in Chapter 10.

Mental health status of centenarians

Cognitive impairment in centenarians is reported with considerable variance, ranging between 34% and 80%. Severe cognitive impairment is estimated to occur in approximately 10% to 40% of this population. Depression, another significant concern, is documented in 13% to 25% of centenarians [Jopp DS, 2016]. The prevalence of depression appears influenced by the centenarians' residence type; institutional living is associated with a higher incidence than those residing at home. Intriguingly, the Sydney Centenarians Study highlighted that centenarians generally reported higher life satisfaction than younger age groups. This observation may stem from their adaptive response to the gradual decline in physical functionality typically experienced with advanced age [Cheng A *et al.*, 2019].

Centenarians' cognitive ability was evaluated with a questionnaire called the Korean Mini-Mental State Examination (K-MMSE). In 2018, centenarians' cognitive ability score was 13.5 points for males and 8.5 points for females, which was higher for males. This tends to be similar to the results known that women have a higher prevalence of dementia than men, but it is thought that there may be a difference from the actual prevalence of cognitive impairment because the cognitive ability score by the questionnaire evaluation

Table 7-1. Comparison of mental health of centenarians between 2001 and 2018

	2001			2018		
	Total	Men	Women	Total	Men	Women
Age	102.3 (100–112)	101.8	102.4	101.8 (100–107)	102	101.7
Sex, n(%)	72	5(7.0)	67(93.0)	37	6(16.2)	31(83.8)
Mental status	N=26			N=37		
K-MMSE	11.0	14.7	7.5	9.63	13.5	8.5
GDS-K	8.26			2.8	2.7	2.8

is affected by the level of education or hearing status. However, compared to centenarians' cognitive ability score in 2001 using the same questionnaire, men (14.7 points) and women (7.5 points) showed almost similar results compared to the 2018 survey(Table 7-1).

In 2018, when centenarians' cognitive ability was analyzed by degree, it was found that most of them needed dementia evaluation, with 7.4% normal, 22.2% mild cognitive impairment, and 70.4% moderate cognitive impairment. Given that 5.6% of centenarians were diagnosed with dementia or receiving treatment in the medical history survey, it suggests that although they have some degree of cognitive impairment, they do not receive active diagnosis or treatment, accepting it as a process of aging. It has been reported that 34-80% of centenarians have a cognitive impairment, and severe cognitive impairment is reported in 10-40% [Jopp DS *et al.*, 2016].

Centenarians' average depression score in 2018 was 2.8 points, which was significantly lower than centenarians' average depression score of 8.26 points in 2001, indicating a relatively low level of depressive symptoms. When analyzing the depression scale in detail from the 2018 centenarians survey, 80% of centenarians scored within the normal range, 13.3% exhibited mild depressive symptoms, and 6.7% showed moderate depressive symptoms. The fact that many centenarians showed a normal range on the depression scale is consistent with the result of relatively high subjective health status. It aligns with prior research, indicating that centenarians tend to exhibit relatively good mental health, implying a significant level of resilience in the very old [Bishop AJ *et al.*, 2010; Richmond RL *et al.*, 2011].

Depression in older adults is distinct from typical depressive disorders, often correlating with the physical and social changes accompanying aging. Factors such as increased physical illness, nursing home admission, and the grief stemming from the loss of family and friends can exacerbate depression in this demographic. Further, there's an observed association between depression in older individuals, cognitive impairment, and reduced daily functioning. According to the Georgia Centenarians Study, centenarians may be particularly susceptible to depression, given that age-related functional and cognitive declines are often irreversible [Scheetz LT *et al.*, 2012].

Summary

In the GuGokSunDam centenarian study, centenarians generally perceived their health positively. We analyzed the health status of Korean centenarians in the GuGokSunDam region by comparing data from 2001 to 2018. Notable changes include a decrease in smoking and alcohol consumption over the years. However, there has been an increased dependency on assistance for daily tasks. Female centenarians demonstrated a higher prevalence of dementia. However, the rate of active diagnoses could be influenced by societal acceptance of cognitive decline as a natural part of aging. Additionally, depression levels have significantly decreased between the two study periods. The research emphasizes the need for holistic support for Korea's older adults, ensuring their physical, mental, and emotional well-being.

References

- Araújo L, Teixeira L, Ribeiro O, Paúl C. Objective vs. Subjective Health in Very Advanced Ages: Looking for Discordance in Centenarians. Front Med (Lausanne). 2018;26;5:189.
- Bishop AJ, Martin P, MacDonald M, *et al.* Predicting happiness among centenarians. Gerontology. 2010;56(1):88-92.
- Cheng A, Leung Y, Crawford JD, Harrison F, Sachdev P, Brodaty H. The psychological health of 207 near-centenarians (95-99) and cenenarians from the Sydney Centenarian Study. Aust N Z J Psychiatry. 2019;53(10): 976-988.
- Cicconetti P, Tafaro L, Tedeschi G, Tomolillo MT, Ciotti V, Troisi G, Marigliano V. Lifestyle and cardiovascular aging in centenarians. Arch Gerontol Geriatr Suppl. 2002;8:93-98.
- Evert J, Lawler E, Bogan H, Perls T. Morbidity profiles of centenarians: survivors, delayers, and escapers. J Gerontol A Biol Sci Med Sci 2003; 58(3):232-237.
- Govindaraju D, Atzmon G, Barzilai N. Genetics, lifestyle and longevity: Lessons from centenarians. Appl Transl Genom. 2015;4:23-32.
- Jopp DS, Park MK, Lehrfeld J, Paggi ME. Physical, cognitive, social and mental health in near-centenarians and centenarians living in New York City: findings from the Fordham Centenarian Study. BMC Geriatr 2016; 16:1.
- Ng R, Sutradhar R, Yao Z, Wodchis WP, Rosella LC. Smoking, drinking, diet and physical activity-modifiable lifestyle risk factors and their associations with age to first chronic disease. Int J Epidemiol. 2020 Feb 1; 49(1):113-130.
- Park K *et al.* Korean centenarians: 20 years of change. Koonja Publishing Inc., 2021.
- Park SC. Korean centenarian study. Seoul: Seoul National University Press, 2002.

- Park SC, Lee MS, Kwon IS, Kwak SC, Yeo EJ. Environment and gender influences on the nutritional and health status of Korean centenarians. Asian J Gerontology and Geriatrics. 2008;3(2):75-83.
- Park SC. Comprehensive approach for studying longevity in Korean centenarians. Asian J Gerontol Geriatr 2012;7:33-38.
- Richmond RL, Law J, Kay-Lambkin F. Physical, mental, and cognitive function in a convenience sample of centenarians in Australia. Journal of the American Geriatrics Society. 2011;59(6):1080-1086.
- Scheetz LT, Martin P, Poon LW. Do centenarians have higher levels of depression? Findings from the Georgia Centenarian Study. J Am Geriatr Soc. 2012;60(2):238-242.

Chapter 08

Insights into the Visual Function of Korean Centenarians

Jonghwa Kim and Kyung Chul Yoon

This study presents an in-depth analysis of the visual function of centenarians in Korea. The research, conducted in 2022, explores various aspects of ocular health, including the prevalence of ocular diseases, history of ocular surgery, visual acuity, and visual discomfort. The study's findings are contextualized within the broader landscape of previous research on aging and ocular health. The study aims to contribute valuable insights into the unique challenges and opportunities the centenarian population presents.

Introduction

'If a person is worth a thousand, their eyes are worth eight hundred,' goes a Korean saying. The significance of preserving visual function in centenarians goes beyond mere scientific inquiry. It delves into the heart of living a fulfilling, independent life in one's twilight years. The ability to see and perceive the world around us is intricately linked to our quality of life, shaping our interactions, mobility, and the sheer joy of experiencing the beauty of the world.

This study aims to provide a comprehensive overview of the visual function of centenarians in Korea. Our research conducted in 2022 delves into their ocular health, encompassing factors such as the prevalence of ocular diseases, history of ocular surgery, visual acuity, and visual discomfort. To place our findings in a broader context, we also review and discuss previous studies on aging and ocular health worldwide. This collective knowledge helps illuminate the challenges and opportunities in promoting visual well-being among centenarians.

Previous Studies

Understanding the visual function of centenarians necessitates a broader perspective gleaned from previous research on aging and ocular health. Several key studies have significantly contributed to our understanding of this field: Reidy and colleagues conducted a study among elderly individuals aged 85–100 and reported an 8% prevalence of glaucoma, highlighting the global impact of this ocular disease in the aging population [Reidy *et al.*, 1998]. Klaver and his team reported that 21% of elderly individuals had undergone cataract surgery, underscoring the significance of cataracts among the elderly [Klaver CC *et al.*, 1998]. Sasaki and associates found a 30% prevalence of cataract surgery among elderly individuals, reaffirming the importance of this intervention [Sasaki H *et al.*, 2000]. Mitchell and colleagues reported a 35% rate of cataract surgery among the elderly, emphasizing the widespread need for such procedures [Mitchell P *et al.*, 1997]. Bergman's study established a visual acuity range of approximately 0.4–0.5 as the threshold for functional loss in daily tasks and pleasures [Bergman B *et al.*, 1992]. McCarty and his team demonstrated that mild visual impairment (visual acuity < 0.5) increases the risk of mortality among the elderly by more than two times [McCarty Ca *et al.*, 2001]. Landstrom's study revealed that 78% of the population aged 85 or older experienced improvements in their ability to perform daily living activities after cataract surgery [Landstrom M *et al.*, 2002]. Birgitta and colleagues reported that more than three-quarters of individuals who underwent cataract surgery maintained a visual acuity of 0.5 or higher at the age of 82 [Birgitta B *et al.*, 2004].

Findings from the 2022 GuGokSunDam Centenarian Study

Our study, conducted in 2022, focused on centenarians in GuGokSunDam area and meticulously examined various facets of their visual function:

Visual function status

In terms of the visual function status among the total subjects aged 95 or older, a notable proportion had undergone ocular surgeries(Table 8-1). Specifically, 5 subjects (6.9%) had undergone cataract surgery, while a significant majority, consisting of 28 subjects (38.9%), had undergone glaucoma surgery. Additionally, 3 subjects (4.2%) had undergone other types of ocular surgeries. None had a history of dry eye diagnosis, though one subject (1.4%) reported experiencing symptoms of dryness or irritation. The diagnoses of ocular diseases within this group revealed a prevalence

Table 8-1. Visual function status in centenarians in Korea.

Category	Total subjects		Aged 100 or older	
	Frequency	Percentage	Frequency	Percentage
History of surgery (n=72)	32	44.4	7	43.8
Glaucoma	5	6.9	0	0
Cataract	28	38.9	6	37.5
Strabismus	0	0	0	0
Blepharoptosis	0	0	0	0
Retinal surgery	0	0	0	0
Refractive surgery (LASIK, LASEK, AK, etc.)	0	0	0	0
Other	3	4.2	1	6.3
Dry eye				
Diagnosis (n=72)	0	0	0	0
Symptoms of dryness or irritation (n=72)	1	1.4	0	0
Diagnosis of cataract (n=72)	26	36.1	5	31.3
Diagnosis of age-related macular degeneration (n=72)	0	0	0	0
Diagnosis of glaucoma (n=72)	5	6.9	0	0

of 36.1% (26 subjects) for cataracts and 6.9% (5 subjects) for glaucoma.

Visual acuity

Visual acuity assessment in this study employed the Han-Cheon-Suk visual acuity chart, a 3-meter Snellen chart, with the measurement results categorized into three distinct groups based on participants' ability to read letters of varying sizes. Among the total subjects aged 95 or older, the distribution of visual acuity in the better eye revealed a diverse range of capabilities(Table 8-2). Approximately

Table 8-2. Visual acuity of a better eye in centenarians in Korea.

Category	Total subjects		Aged 100 or older	
	Frequency	Percentage	Frequency	Percentage
〈0.02	1	1.8	0	0
0.02-0.2	16	28.6	5	50
0.3-0.5	26	46.4	4	40
〉0.5	7	12.5	1	10

1.8% (1 subject) of the subjects demonstrated visual acuity levels below 0.02, rendering them unable to read large letters. About 28.6% (15 subjects) of the participants exhibited visual acuity ranging from 0.02 to 0.2, enabling them to read large letters. A substantial proportion, approximately 46.4% (26 subjects), fell within the visual acuity range of 0.3 to 0.5, signifying their capacity to read medium-sized letters. Moreover, 12.5% (7 subjects) displayed visual acuity greater than 0.5, indicating their ability to read small letters.

Regarding reported visual discomfort, the majority of the subjects, comprising 86.2% (50 subjects) of the total, indicated that they experienced no visual discomfort during the assessment. Approximately 12.1% (7 subjects) reported feeling somewhat uncomfortable, while only a single subject, accounting for 1.7% of the cohort, reported feeling very uncomfortable.

These findings offer valuable insights into the distribution of visual acuity and the prevalence of visual discomfort among individuals aged 95 or older in the study, shedding light on the varying degrees of visual function within this population.

Discussion

Among the diseases related to visual function, cataracts showed the highest prevalence (36.1% in 95 years of age or older and 31.3% in 100 years of age or older) and glaucoma showed the second highest prevalence (6.9% in 95 years of age or older). In similar studies from other countries, the prevalence of glaucoma was reported to be 8% among elderly people aged 85–100 [Reidy *et al.*, 1998].

Regarding cataracts, which was reported to be the most common visual function related disease in this study, previous studies from other countries targeting older people reported various percentages of those who underwent cataract surgery [21%; Klaver CC *et al.*, 1998; 30%: Sasaki H *et al.*, 2000; 35%: Mitchell P *et al.*, 1997]. In this study, the percentage of patients who underwent cataract surgery was 38.9% (95 years or older) and 37.5% (100 years or older), showing similar or slightly higher results compared to previous reports.

At the age of 82, visual acuity of approximately 0.4–0.5 is known to be the threshold to functional loss in daily tasks and pleasures [Bergman B *et al.*, 1992]. In addition, it has been reported that mild visual impairment (visual acuity less than 0.5) increases the risk of death in the elderly by more than two times [McCarty C *et al.*, 2001). Furthermore, it has been reported that 78% of the population aged 85 or older experienced an improvement in difficulty in performing activities of daily living after cataract surgery [Landstrom M *et al.*, 2002]. Another study targeting elderly people reported that more than three-quarters of those who underwent cataract surgery maintained a visual acuity of 0.5 or higher at the age of 82 [Birgitta B *et al.*, 2004]. Therefore, proper visual function management, including cataract surgery, in older people is essential for prolonging survival.

Visual impairment increases with age. 35.5% of the population over 85 of age complained of visual impairment [van der Pols JC *et al.*, 2000]. Another study in people over the age of 70 reported that visual acuity began to deteriorate at the age of 44 and decreased by about one-third by the age of 88 [Sjostrand J *et al.*, 2011]. In this study, 12.5% (95 years of age or older) and 10.0% (100 years of age or older) had visual acuity of 0.5 or higher, showing similar rates in both groups. Most subjects were distributed in the 0.02–0.5 interval where they could read large and middle-sized letters (75.0% at 95 years of age or older and 90.0% at 100 years of age or older). However, 86.2% (95 years of age or older) and 93.8% (100 years of age or older) did not complain of visual discomfort, which is thought to reflect the characteristics of the rural lifestyle in the survey area.

Therefore, based on the comprehensive visual function test results, it is recommended to monitor and manage visual function and perform appropriate procedures, including cataract surgery, to ensure prolonged survival and an improved quality of life in older people.

Summary

Through the analysis of the visual acuity and eye health of centenarians in GuGokSunDam area of South Korea, this study has demonstrated that, with proper care and management, the degree of visual impairment is not significantly worse compared to the general population. This research underscores the importance of ophthalmic examinations and the necessity for appropriate interventions such as cataract surgery and treatments for other ocular diseases.

PART III

References

- Bergman B, Weinreb RN. The threshold visual field. Acta Ophthalmol. 1992;70(5):709-715.
- Birgitta B, Carl-Gustaf L. Visual acuity in 82-year-olds: Relationship to medical, psychological and social factors. *Acta Ophthalmologica*. 2004; 82(5):345-350.
- Klaver CC, Wolfs RC, Vingerling JR, Hofman A, de Jong PT. Age-specific prevalence and causes of blindness and visual impairment in an older population: The Rotterdam Study. *Arch Ophthalmol.* 1998;116(5):653-658.
- Landstrom M, Lundstrom M, Stenevi U, Thorburn W. Visual function and quality of life in patients treated for cataract in one eye: A prospective cross-sectional study. *Acta Ophthalmol.* 2002;80(5):507-511.
- McCarty CA, Nanjan MB, Taylor HR. Vision impairment predicts 5 year mortality. *Br J Ophthalmol.* 2001;85(5):322-326.
- Mitchell P, Cumming RG, Attebo K, Panchapakesan J. Prevalence of cataract in Australia: The Blue Mountains Eye Study. *Ophthalmology.* 1997;104(5): 581-588.
- Reidy P, Smith D, Kirchner E, *et al.* Prevalence of glaucoma in an Australian urban population. *BMJ.* 1998;312(5):22-24.
- Sasaki H, Jonasson F, Jonsson V, *et al.* Prevalence of age-related maculopathy in old age. The Reykjavik Eye Study. Ophthalmologica. 2000;214(5):235-238.

Chapter 09

The Auditory Function of Korean Centenarians

Sungsu Lee and Hyong-Ho Cho

Introduction

Hearing loss can have significant effects on elderly people, impacting their overall quality of life in various ways. Hearing loss can make it challenging for elderly individuals to communicate effectively with family members, friends, and healthcare professionals. This can lead to feelings of isolation and frustration. Elderly individuals may avoid social gatherings, which can contribute to loneliness and depression. Hearing loss can lead to a reduced overall quality of life. It can impact an individual's ability to enjoy hobbies, participate in activities, and maintain relationships with loved ones.

In the current chapter, influence of the auditory function on health of elderly population will be reviewed. Status of centenarians and near-centenarians through GuGokSunDam study will be discussed.

Methods in GuGokSunDam Study for Hearing Threshold and Condition Related to Hearing Loss

Participant and hearing threshold measurement

Total 74 participants (age 95-109; mean 98.2 years) were enrolled in the study. There were 17 males and 57 females. Pure tone audiometry was checked to evaluate the hearing threshold using a tablet-based device and a headset. Four frequencies of 500, 1000, 2000, 4000 Hz were measured in the pure tone hearing test(Figure 9-1). Average hearing threshold was calculated as follows; (500Hz + 2x1000Hz + 2x2000Hz + 4000Hz) / 6

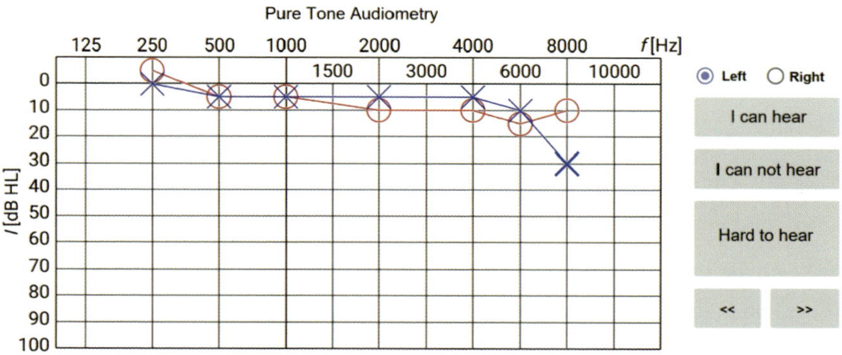

Figure 9-1. Tablet based pure tone audiometry. Air conduction hearing thresholds were measured in frequencies from 250Hz to 8000Hz. Red circle marks indicate right side, blue 'x' marks indicate left side thresholds.

Lifestyle habits and hearing ability survey

Lifestyle habits were investigated through the following questionnaires(Table 9-1, 9-2, 9-3). Korean hearing handicap inventory in elderly(K-HHIE) was modified from the original version(Table 9-3).

The survey was conducted by narrowing down 10 questions from the original 25 (modified K-HHIE). Total score ranged from 0～40 (10 × 4) instead of 0～100 (25 × 4).

Table 9-1. Health status and lifestyle survey

8. Do you usually use hearing aids?
(1) Use (2) Do not use

9. When talking on the phone or having a conversation with the person next to you, how can you hear the other person's voice?
(If you use a hearing aid, please tell us based on the condition in which you are wearing the hearing aid.)
(1) Very good (2) Good (3) Bad (4) Very bad

10. Are you currently having trouble doing your daily activities because of your hearing?
(1) Yes (2) No

11. Have you ever smoked?
(1) I have never smoked (☞ To question 12)
(2) I smoked in the past, but I don't smoke now.
(3) Currently smoking
11-1. Current period: years months
11-2. Current smoking amount: cigarettes/day

Table 9-2. Examination of vision, hearing, and chewing function

2. Hearing Function

2-1. Do you use hearing aids (hearing aids)?
(1) Yes
(2) No

2-2. When it comes to phone calls or having conversations with the person next to you, how much inconvenience does your hearing cause in your daily life?
(1) It is not uncomfortable
(2) It's uncomfortable
(3) Very uncomfortable

Table 9-3. Modified Korean hearing handicap inventory for elderly (K-HHIE)

	0	2	4
1. Do you have trouble meeting new people because you have hearing loss?			
2. Do you feel frustrated when talking to your family because you are hard of hearing?			
3. Can't you hear when others whisper quietly?			
4. Do you feel disabled due to hearing problems?			
5. Do you have trouble visiting friends or neighbors because you are hard of hearing?			
6. Do you have difficulty participating in religious events due to hearing loss?			
7. Do you sometimes get into fights with your family because you are hard of hearing?			
8. Are you having trouble listening to television or radio?			
9. Do you feel that your hearing problems are limiting your personal or social life?			
10. Do you have trouble conversing when you're at a restaurant with friends because you're hard of hearing?			
Total Score	0 ~ 40		

Findings and Discussion

Aspects of hearing loss on health in elderly people and centenarian

• Prevalence hearing loss in elderly population

According to the World Health Organization [WHO, 2021], nearly 1.5 billion people have hearing impairment and it is estimated that 2.5 billion people (1 in 4) will have hearing loss by 2050. Of these, at least 700 million are expected to need hearing care and rehabilitation.

According to a report by the Korean Society of Otolaryngology, the prevalence of age-related hearing loss in the population aged 65 or older is approximately 38% in Korea. This means that two out of five elderly people suffer from hearing loss. The number of patients visiting hospitals due to age-related hearing loss (patients in their 60s or older) has also increased rapidly, with the number of 46% increment in 2021 compared to 2017 (Korea Health Insurance

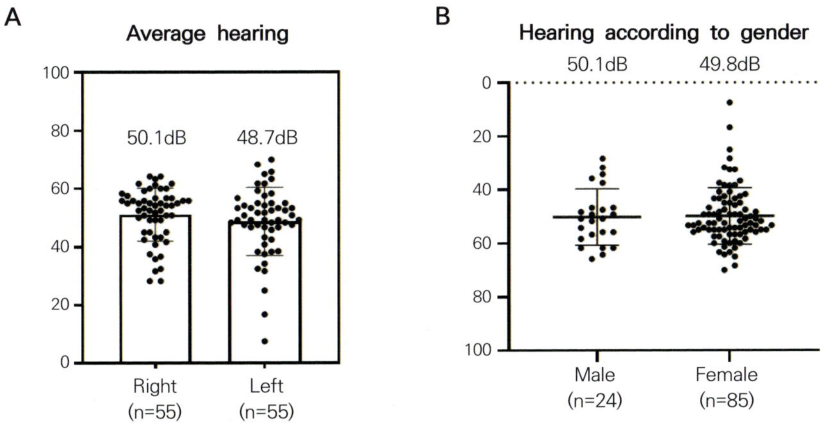

Figure 9-2. Average hearing level of total participants (centenarians and near-centenarians). There was no difference between left and right ears (A). Hearing threshold was comparable between males and females (B).

Table 9-4. Hearing levels according in centenarians and near-centenarians

Category	Near centenarians (n=45)		Centenarians (n=11)	
	Frequency	%	Frequency	%
Normal	0	0	0	0
Mild HL (≥26dB)	9	20	2	18
Moderate (≥41dB)	27	40	5	46
Moderate-Severe (≥56dB)	9	20	4	36
Severe (≥71dB)	0	0	0	0
Profound (≥91dB)	0	0	0	0

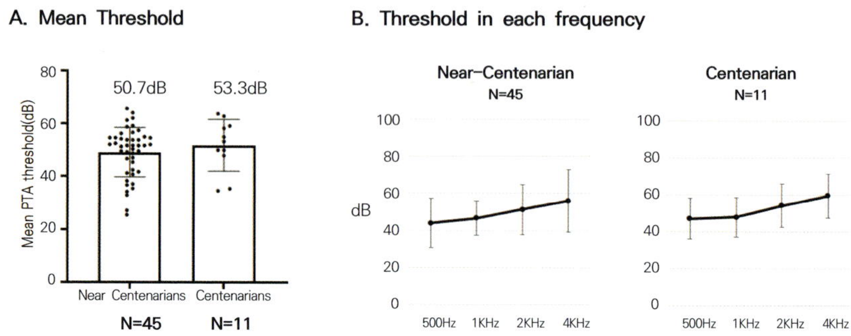

Figure 9-3. Hearing thresholds between centenarians and near-centenarians. mean hearing (A) and average hearing level of each frequency (B) were similar between centenarians and near-centenarians.

Review & Assessment Service).

In GuGokSunDam study, average hearing threshold in centenarians and near-centenarians was around 50dB. There was no difference between left and right ear. Interestingly, there was also no difference between male and female participants(Figure 9-2B). Hearing level was comparable between centenarians and near-centenarians(Table 9-4, Figure 9-3A and 9-3B) in all pure tone frequencies.

- **Effect of hearing loss and daily life in elderly**

Hearing loss can pose safety risks for the elderly, as they may not hear important sounds, such as alarms, sirens, or approaching vehicles. This can increase the likelihood of accidents and falls. Untreated hearing loss may have indirect health consequences, as it can lead to stress, sleep disturbances, and reduced overall well-being. In centenarians and near-centenarians, speech understanding was limited in 2/3 of the total participants. Daily activities were limited in 71%(Figure 9-4). Hearing handicap inventory was significantly higher in patients with more severe hearing loss(Figure 9-5).

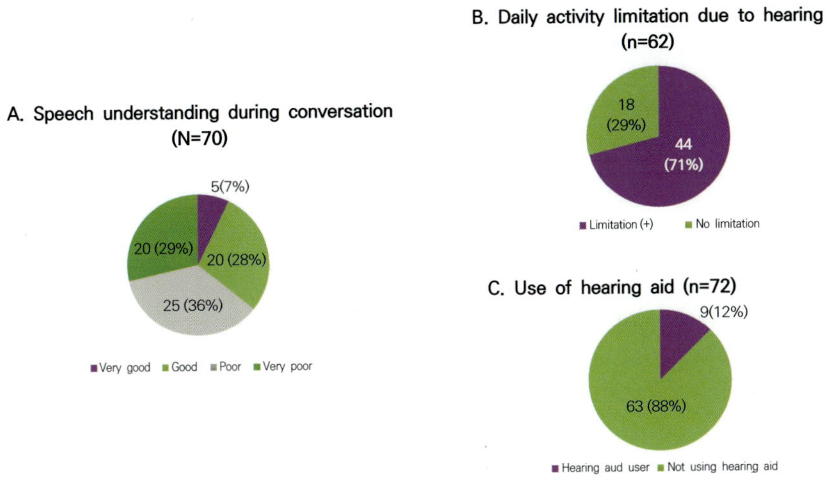

Figure 9-4. Hearing lifestyle and health status. Speech understanding was limited in 2/3 of the total centenarians and near-centenarians (A). Daily activities were limited in 71% (B). Hearing rehabilitation using hearing aids was only seen in 12% of the participants (C).

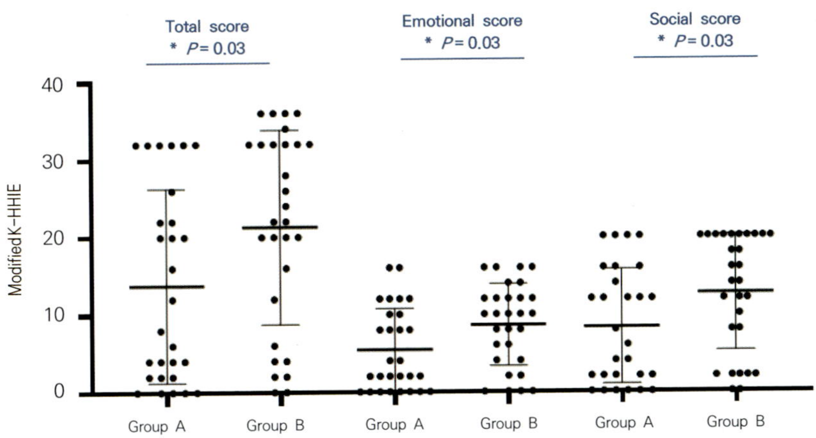

Figure 9-5. Modified Korean hearing handicap inventory in elderly (K-HHIE) scores according to hearing levels. Group A is a group with less than moderate hearing loss(〈 41dB) on one ear and less than moderate-severe hearing loss (〈 56dB) on the other side. Group B is more than moderate hearing loss on one ear and more than moderate-severe hearing loss on the other side. Group B participant showed significantly higher K-HHIE score compared to group A scores (p 〈 0.05)

- Influence of hearing loss on cognitive impairment and dementia

Hearing loss can have a significant impact on cognitive function and may be associated with an increased risk of dementia. There have been several reports on the possible pathomechanism how [Griffiths TM. *et al.*, 2020] hearing loss can affect cognitive function and contribute to dementia. First, is the Cognitive Load. When individuals have hearing loss, their brains must work harder to process and understand speech and environmental sounds. This increased cognitive load can lead to mental fatigue, making it more challenging to focus on other cognitive tasks. Over time, this added cognitive effort can contribute to cognitive decline. Secondly, Hearing loss can lead to social isolation and withdrawal from social activities. This isolation can result in reduced cognitive stimulation and opportunities for social interaction, both of which are important for maintaining cognitive function. Loneliness and social isolation have been linked to an increased risk of cognitive decline and dementia. Thirdly, Hearing loss can make it difficult to communicate effectively with others. This can lead to frustration, anxiety, and a decreased willingness to engage in conversations or participate in social activities. Reduced communication can impact cognitive skills related to language and comprehension. There also have been studies showing that untreated hearing loss may be associated with changes in brain structure. Brain regions responsible for processing sound may atrophy over time if they are not sufficiently stimulated. These structural changes can have implications for cognitive function.

It's important to note that while there is evidence linking hearing loss to cognitive decline and dementia, more research is needed to fully understand the mechanisms and causality of this relationship. However, managing hearing loss through interventions such as hearing aids or cochlear implants can potentially mitigate some of these cognitive impacts [Dawes P. *et al.*, 2015] and improve overall quality of life for individuals with hearing loss

- **Hearing loss and lifespan mortality**

There have been several reports inclining that hearing loss in the elderly population can increase mortality through various mechanisms. Several studies have shown a strong link between untreated hearing loss in older adults and increased social isolation and loneliness. A lack of social engagement and support networks can contribute to depression and anxiety, which are known risk factors for mortality [Mick P. *et al.,* 2014]. Multiple studies have suggested a connection between hearing loss and cognitive decline in older adults. Cognitive impairment and dementia are associated with higher mortality rates [Lin FR, 2011]. Hearing loss can compromise safety, making older adults more vulnerable to accidents and injuries, which can have fatal consequences. Difficulty hearing alarms, sirens, or warnings in emergency situations may result in adverse outcomes [Strawbridge WJ *et al.*, 2000].

Elderly individuals with hearing loss may experience challenges in accessing healthcare services, receiving medical advice, or adhering to treatment plans. These barriers can lead to unmanaged health conditions, potentially impacting mortality rates [Wallhagen MI, 2010].

Hearing loss can contribute to mental health issues, including depression and anxiety, which have been associated with increased mortality rates in older adults [Contrera KJ, 2017].

It is important to recognize that hearing loss often coexists with other age-related health conditions, making it challenging to isolate its specific impact on mortality. However, research consistently suggests that addressing hearing loss through interventions like hearing aids and cochlear implants, as well as promoting social engagement and mental health support, can potentially reduce mortality risks in the elderly population.

- **Hearing rehabilitation in elderly patients**

Hearing aid users in centerarian and near-centararian were equally about 12%(Figure 9-6). Hearing rehabilitation is crucial for the elderly population with hearing loss because it can significantly improve their quality of life, mental well-being, and overall health. Hearing rehabilitation, which may include the use of hearing aids or cochlear implants, can improve an elderly person's ability to communicate effectively with family, friends, and healthcare providers. This helps reduce feelings of isolation and frustration associated with hearing loss. Improved hearing allows individuals to engage in social activities, which can stimulate the brain and support cognitive health. Treating hearing loss can alleviate feelings of depression and anxiety, which are common among older adults with hearing impairment. Better emotional well-being positively impacts an individual's overall quality of life. Hearing aids and other assistive devices can enhance safety by allowing individuals to hear important auditory cues, such as alarms, sirens, and warnings. This can help prevent accidents and injuries. Hearing aids are commonly used to amplify sounds for individuals with mild to moderate hearing loss. Properly fitted and adjusted hearing aids can make a significant difference in hearing ability. For individuals with severe or profound hearing loss who do not benefit from hearing aids, cochlear implants may be an option. These devices can restore a sense of sound by directly stimulating the auditory nerve. Assistive listening devices, such as amplified phones and TV listening systems, can be used to improve hearing in specific situations. Support groups and counseling can help individuals and their families cope with the emotional and social challenges of hearing loss in elderly people. Elderly individuals and their caregivers should learn effective communication strategies, such as speaking clearly, facing the person, and minimizing background noise. It is also important to regularly perform hearing assessments by an audiologist. This can help monitor hearing loss progression and adjust treatment accordingly.

Hearing rehabilitation should be personalized to the individual's needs and preferences. Consulting with an audiologist or hearing healthcare professional is essential for a comprehensive evaluation and tailored rehabilitation plan. It's important to recognize that hearing loss is a common age-related issue, and effective interventions can significantly enhance the overall well-being of elderly individuals with hearing impairment.

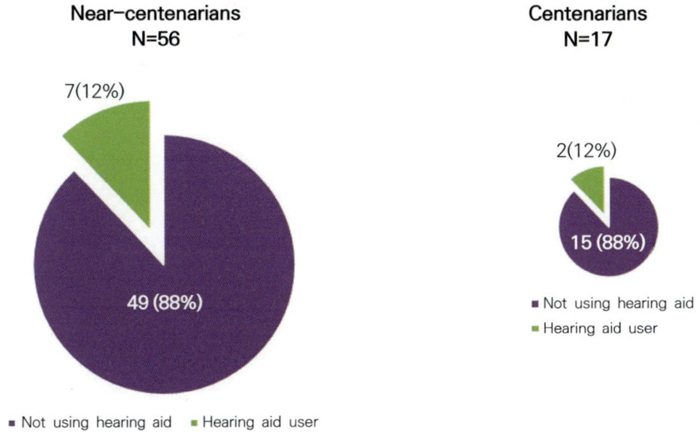

Figure 9-6. Hearing aid users between centenarians and near-centenarians. The proportion of hearing aid users was exactly the same between both groups.

Summary

Hearing impairment is one of the most common sensory deficit, especially in elderly population. The hearing threshold was around 50dB centenarian and near-centenarian through Gogoksundam survey. Hearing loss can cause social isolation and reduced daily activity. This accelerates cognitive decline and dementia. Moreover, it can increase mortality. Further studies are yet to be done to reveal the exact mechanism of this adverse effect of hearing loss. It is important to encourage elderly or to participate in auditory rehabilitation such as hearing aid, cochlear implantation.

PART III

References

- Contrera KJ, Sung YK, Betz J, Li L, Lin FR. Change in loneliness after intervention with cochlear implants or hearing aids. Laryngoscope. 2017; 127(8):1885-1889.
- Dawes P, Emsley R, Cruickshanks KJ, Moore DR, Fortnum H, Edmondson-Jones M, McCormack A, Munro KJ. Plos One 2015;10(3):e0119616
- Griffiths TM, Lad M, Kumar S, Holmes E, McMurray B, Maguire EA, Billig AJ, Sedley W. How can hearing loss cause dementia? Neuron 2020; 108(3):401-412.
- Lin FR. Hearing loss and cognition among older adults in the United States. J Gerontol A Biol Sci Med Sci. 2011;66(10):1131-1136.
- Mick P, Kawachi I, Lin FR. The association between hearing loss and social isolation in older adults. Otolaryngol Head Neck Surg. 2014;150(3): 378-384.
- Strawbridge WJ, Wallhagen MI, Shema SJ, Kaplan GA. Negative consequences of hearing impairment in old age: a longitudinal analysis. Gerontologist. 2000;40(3):320-326.
- Wallhagen MI. The stigma of hearing loss. Gerontologist. 2010;50(1):66-75.
- WHO: 1 in 4 people projected to have hearing problems by 2050. Available at: https://www.who.int/news/item/02-03-2021-who-1-in-4-people-projected-to-have-hearing-problems-by-2050

Chapter 10

Lifestyle Changes of Korean Centenarians

Ki-Hong Kim and Jae-Young Han

For the past 20 years, the lives and lifestyles of Koreans have undergone many changes. These changes can be attributed to income improvement, science and technology development, telecommunication, and social culture flow. Income levels have increased due to economic growth, which considerably improved the quality of life. Through this, we have invested in housing, education, medical care, and leisure activities. Advanced technology has vastly increased the amount of accessible information and services. With the development of communication technology, we can effortlessly contact each other, and with the development of transportation technology, the entire nation is within a day's reach. Along with the advancement of medical technology, we can hope to live longer, happier, and healthier. These lifestyle changes have greatly influenced older adults and are also thought to have influenced centenarians in many ways. In this chapter, we will find out how the lifestyles of the centenarians have changed compared to previous studies.

Lifestyle Habits of Centenarians

We examined centenarians' lifestyle habits regarding sleep duration, alcohol usage, and smoking. The average sleep duration of centenarians was confirmed to be 8.88 hours per day. It is understood that centenarians have a relatively regulated life and did not show much difference from the 9 hours in 2001. There was also no gender difference. Based on this, it can be interpreted that sufficient sleep of over 8 hours is a significant factor in becoming a centenarian (Table 10-1).

It was demonstrated that centenarians' smoking rate and alcohol consumption rate decreased overall compared to 2001. There is currently 1 (2.8%) centenarian smoker, a significant decrease compared to 9 (13%) in 2001. The rate of those with past smoking experience has also decreased to 1 in 4 people compared to result of 2001 of 1 in 3 people. Comparing the 2018 sex difference in past smoking experience rates showed a rate of 83.3% for men and 13.3% for women, indicating a higher number for men than women.

The alcohol consumption rate of centenarians also decreased significantly. Centenarians currently consuming alcohol in 2018 is only 6.1%, a great reduction from 85% in 2001 (Table 10-2).

Table 10-1. **Centenarian's sleep duration** (From Park K *et al.* Korean centenarians: 20 years of change. Koonja Publishing Inc.; 2021, with permission)

	2001	2018					
	Age 100 and over (n=72)	Age 100 and over (n=37)			Age 95 and over (n=98)		
		Total	Men	Women	Total	Men	Women
Sleep duration	9.0	8.88	8.40	9.00	8.69	8.08	8.76

Table 10-2. **Centenarian's alcohol consumption rate and smoking rate** (From Park K *et al.* Korean centenarians: 20 years of change. Koonja Publishing Inc.; 2021, with permission)

		2001	2018					
		Age 100 and over (n=72)	Age 100 and over (37)			Age 95 and over (98)		
			Total	Men	Women	Total	Men	Women
Smoking	No smoking experience	48(66.0)	27(75.0)	1(16.7)	26(86.7)	68(70.8)	4(25.0)	64(80.0)
	Smoking experience	24(34.0)	9(25.0)	5(83.3)	4(13.3)	28(29.2)	12(75.0)	16(20.0)
	Currently smoking	9(13.0)	1(2.8)	0(0)	1(3.3)	5(5.2)	0(0)	5(6.3)
	Currently not smoking	15(21.0)	8(89.0)	5(83.3)	3(10.0)	23(24.0)	12(75.0)	11(13.7)
Alcohol consumption	Current alcohol consumption	12(85.0)	2(6.1)	1(16.7)	1(3.7)	9(9.7)	5(31.3)	4(5.2)
	Current alcohol abstinence	2(15.0)	31(93.9)	5(83.3)	26(96.3)	84(90.3)	11(68.8)	73(94.8)

* Missing values due to item nonresponse

Social Characteristics of Centenarians

To examine centenarians' social characteristics, we investigated their activity range or duration, the degree to which they socialize, the reasons for not socializing, and the degree and gathering participation.

In 2001, the centenarians' activity range was highest for staying within their rooms (37.5%). Nonetheless, in the 2018 survey, the percentage of centenarians staying within their rooms is 21.2%, 16.3% including near-centenarians, which is relatively lower. Rather, the number of cases in which their activity range extended to within the house, the neighborhood, the village, and even not too far out of the village, and working in the fields have increased. With a more comprehensive look, the percentage of centenarians who are sedentary or stay within their rooms has decreased (37.5% in 2001 → 21.2% in 2018), and the number of centenarians who stay within their house (25.0% in 2001 → 33.3% in 2018), within the neighborhood or the village (16.7% in 2001 → 24.2% in 2018), as well as not too far out of the village and working in the fields (16.7% in 2001 → 21.2% in 2018) has increased. An examination of the 2018 survey for gender differences shows that Men centenarians have a larger activity range than women centenarians(Table 10-3).

It is speculated that this increase in active centenarians is due to the advancement of medical and welfare services compared with 20 years ago.

Compared to 2001, the 2018 survey additionally examined activity duration, the degree to which they socialize, and gatherings. The results are as such. With regards to activity duration, most centenarians were shown to be active for 30 min to under 1 hour.

Table 10-3. Centenarian's range of activity (From Park K *et al.* Korean centenarians: 20 years of change. Koonja Publishing Inc.; 2021, with permission)

	2001	2018					
	Age 100 and over (n=72)	Age 100 and over (n=37)			Age 95 and over (n=98)		
		Total	Men	Women	Total	Men	Women
Within room	27(37.5)	7(21.2)	1(16.7)	6(22.2)	15(16.3)	1(6.3)	14(18.4)
Within house	18(25.0)	11(33.3)	2(33.3)	9(33.3)	33(35.9)	6(37.5)	27(35.5)
Within the neighborhood and village	15(20.8)	8(24.2)	1(16.7)	7(26.0)	27(29.3)	4(25.0)	23(30.3)
Not too far out of the village/fieldwork	12(16.7)	7(21.2)	2(33.3)	5(18.5)	17(18.5)	5(31.3)	12(15.8)

* Missing values due to item nonresponse

Table 10-4. **Centenarian's range of activity duration** (From Park K *et al.* Korean centenarians: 20 years of change. Koonja Publishing Inc.; 2021, with permission)

		2018					
		Age 100 and over (n=37)			Age 95 and over (n=98)		
		Total	Men	Women	Total	Men	Women
Activity duration	Almost never	12(33.3)	1(16.7)	11(36.7)	23(24.0)	1(6.3)	22(27.5)
	Below 30 min	6(16.7)	1(16.7)	5(16.7)	27(28.1)	5(31.3)	22(27.5)
	30 min - below 1 hour	13(36.1)	3(50.0)	10(33.3)	29(30.2)	5(31.3)	24(30.0)
	1 hour - below 2 hours	4(11.1)	0(0)	4(13.3)	16(16.7)	4(25.0)	12(15.0)
	2 hours - below 3 hours	0(0)	0(0)	0(0)	0(0)	0(0)	0(0)
	3 hours or more	1(2.8)	1(16.7)	0(0)	1(1.0)	1(6.3)	0(0)

* Missing values due to item nonresponse

Approximately 7 out of 10 centenarians are active for over 30 min, and when near-centenarians are included, the activity duration increases. In a sex comparison, it was found that men tended to be a little more active than women(Table 10-4).

Table 10-5. **The degree of socialization** (From Park K *et al.* Korean centenarians: 20 years of change. Koonja Publishing Inc.; 2021, with permission)

	2018					
	Age 100 and over (n=37)			Age 95 and over (n=98)		
	Total	Men	Women	Total	Men	Women
Socialize often	16(44.4)	3(50.0)	13(43.3)	36(37.5)	7(43.8)	29(36.3)
Socialize on special occasions	2(5.6)	0(0)	2(6.7)	5(5.2)	0(0)	5(6.3)
Do not socialize well	18(50.0)	3(50.0)	15(50.0)	55(57.3)	9(56.3)	46(57.5)

* Missing values due to item nonresponse

An examination of the degree to which centenarians socialize showed that half of the centenarians often socialize on special occasions, while the rest do not socialize well. There were no significant sex differences found(Table 10-5).

As a result of examining why the centenarians responded that they did not socialize well, the most common reason was "because they are physically unwell." Some responded, "I would like to socialize, but there have been no opportunities or companions."(Table 10-6) This implies that the percentage of those who socialize is more likely to increase with better physical health.

Next, we investigated the degree of gathering participation in centenarians. Most of those 100 and over and 40% of those 95 and over participated in gatherings. Even at 40%, it is still very encouraging that centenarians participate in group gatherings and social activities. There are several cases in which they have participated in the past but are currently not partaking in the gatherings. As examined beforehand, this could be attributed to health issues or having no gatherings to engage in.

Table 10-6. **Reasons for not socializing well** (From Park K *et al.* Korean centenarians: 20 years of change. Koonja Publishing Inc.; 2021, with permission)

	2018					
	Age 100 and over (n=37)			Age 95 and over (n=98)		
	Total	Men	Women	Total	Men	Women
Would like to, but no opportunities/companions	3(17.6)	1(33.3)	2(14.3)	5(9.4)	2(25.0)	3(6.7)
Too bothersome	1(5.9)	0(0)	1(7.1)	3(5.7)	0(0)	3(6.7)
Physically unwell to socialize	9(52.9)	1(33.3)	8(57.1)	35(66.0)	4(50.0)	31(68.9)
Others	4(23.5)	1(33.3)	3(21.4)	10(18.9)	2(25.0)	8(17.8)

* Others: taciturn, no interest, recently relocated

With a focus on the respondents who participate in gatherings, more than half the locations were senior citizen centers (senior halls), and there were other various locations such as nursing homes, daycare centers, neighboring houses, and religious institutions. It can be argued that this result reaffirms the importance of citizen centers and senior halls as gathering sites for older adults(Table 10-7).

Table 10-7. **Degree of gathering participation and gathering locations** (From Park K *et al.* Korean centenarians: 20 years of change. Koonja Publishing Inc.; 2021, with permission)

		2018					
		Age 100 and over			Age 95 and over		
		Total	Men	Women	Total	Men	Women
Degree of gathering participation	Participates	15(55.5)	1(25.0)	14(70.0)	32(40.5)	5(38.5)	27(40.9)
	Past participation, no current participation	9(33.3)	3(75.0)	5(25.0)	79(46.8)	8(61.5)	29(43.9)
	Never participated	1(4.2)	0(0)	1(5.0)	10(12.7)	0(0)	10(15.2)
Gathering locations	Senior citizen center (senior halls)	8(53.3)	1(100.0)	7(50.0)	22(68.8)	4(80.0)	18(66.7)
	Religious institutions	1(6.7)	0(0)	1(7.1)	2(6.3)	0(0)	2(7.4)
	Nursing homes	3(20.0)	0(0)	3(21.4)	4(12.5)	0(0)	4(14.8)
	Daycare centers	1(6.7)	0(0)	1(7.1)	2(6.3)	1(20.0)	1(3.7)
	Neighboring houses	2(13.3)	0(0)	2(14.3)	2(6.3)	0(0)	2(7.4)

Degree of gathering participation respondents: 24 from age 100 and over, 79 from age 95 and over. Gathering locations respondents: Of those who responded to the degree of gathering participation, 15 from age 100 and over, 32 from age 95 and over.

Allowing centenarians to maintain good health while providing and managing places where older adults can easily gather, such as senior citizens' halls, nursing homes, and daycare centers, will enable them to partake in social gatherings with the people nearby. By such means, the centenarians can steadily establish social relationships with those around them.

Lifestyle Examined by Activities of Daily Living

During senescence, it gradually becomes difficult to conduct daily life activities alone due to the deterioration of physical or cognitive functions caused by frailty. In such cases, there comes a time when the help of those around you becomes a necessity. It can be said that with extremely senior individuals such as centenarians, specific diseases' presence or absence are important. Nonetheless, the ability to lead an independent life alone may be more significant. The ability to perform activities of daily living is a tool that can evaluate whether one can lead an independent life and is widely used to assess the functional levels of older adults. As for the activities of the daily living questionnaire, there is a Korean version of activities of daily living (K-ADL) and a Korean version of instrumental activities of daily living (K-IADL). Among them, the K-ADL is a tool that evaluates the individual's activity performance necessary to take care of and maintain their body daily, such as bathing, dressing, toileting, transferring, eating, and continence. The other evaluative tool, the K-IADL, assesses items needed for a social life, such as shopping, using the telephone, using public transportation, doing light housework, food preparation, doing the laundry, grooming, and going out short distances. Based on these, we aim to study how the centenarians can independently perform daily and social activities.

Activities of daily living

In the 2001 centenarian study, the assessment of activities of daily life showed that it was relatively possible for centenarian individuals to perform basic activities in the order of toileting at 77.9%, eating at 73.6%, dressing at 72.3%, transferring at 63.9%, and bathing at 45.8%. However, in the 2018 study, all daily life activities declined except for eating at 82.9%, toileting at 65.7%, transferring at 57.1%, dressing at 43.9%, and bathing at 22.9%(Table 10-8).

Table 10-8. Centenarian's activities of daily living (From Park K *et al.* Korean centenarians: 20 years of change. Koonja Publishing Inc.; 2021, with permission)

		2001			2018		
		Age 100 and over (n=72)			Age 100 and over (n=36)		
		Dependent	Slightly dependent	Independent	Dependent	Slightly dependent	Independent
ADL	Bathing	31(43.1)	8(11.1)	33(45.8)	21(60.0)	6(17.1)	8(22.9)
	Dressing	15(20.8)	5(6.9)	52(72.3)	12(34.3)	8(22.9)	15(42.9)
	Toileting	17(23.7)	12(16.7)	56(77.9)	7(20.0)	5(14.3)	23(65.7)
	Transferring	17(23.6)	9(12.5)	46(63.9)	8(22.9)	7(20.2)	20(57.1)
	Eating	6(8.3)	5(6.9)	53(73.6)	2(5.7)	4(11.4)	29(82.9)
	Continence				7(20.0)	1(2.9)	27(77.1)
	Washing face and hand				9(25.7)	8(22.9)	18(51.4)

Table 10-9. **Activities of daily living by household type** (From Park K *et al.* Korean centenarians: 20 years of change. Koonja Publishing Inc.; 2021, with permission)

		2001			2018								
		Age 100 and over (n=72)			Age 100 and over, living alone (n=9)			Age 100 and over, living with family (n=20)			Age 100 and over, facility resident (n=7)		
		Depen dent	Slightly depen dent	Indepen dent	Depen dent	Slightly depen dent	Indepen dent	Depen dent	Slightly depen dent	Indepen dent	Depen dent	Slightly depen dent	Indepen dent
ADL	Bathing	43.1	11.1	45.8	33.3	11.1	55.6	65.0	20.0	15.0	83.3	16.7	0
	Dressing	20.8	6.9	72.3	22.2	11.1	66.7	30.0	30.0	40.0	66.7	16.7	16.7
	Toileting	23.7	16.7	77.9	0	22.2	77.8	15.0	15.0	70.0	66.7	0	33.3
	Trans-ferring	23.6	12.5	63.9	0	11.1	88.9	15.0	30.0	55.0	83.3	0	16.7
	Eating	8.3	6.9	73.6	0	0	100	5.0	15.0	80.0	16.7	16.7	66.7

We were expecting an overall improvement in the results compared to before, but conversely, several examinations were conducted on the cause of this decline. Accordingly, in the 2001 centenarian study nearly 20 years ago, most centenarians lived alone or with family and none were residing in facilities, which proved to be the difference between the 2001 and 2018 surveys. Therefore, a reanalysis was conducted according to household types(Table 10-9). The result showed that the elderly living in facilities often needed full assistance, affecting the statistical analysis.

Instrumental activities of daily living

In the case of instrumental activities of daily living necessary for social life, 2018 centenarians were more likely able to perform all the activities independently compared to 2001 centenarians, unlike the previous results of the activities of daily living(Table

Table 10-10. Centenarian's instrumental activities of daily living (From Park K *et al.* Korean centenarians: 20 years of change. Koonja Publishing Inc.; 2021, with permission)

		2001			2018		
		Age 100 and over (n=72)			Age 100 and over (n=37)		
		Dependent	Slightly dependent	Independent	Dependent	Slightly dependent	Independent
IADL	Shopping	58(80.6)	10(13.9)	4(5.6)	28(80.0)	3(8.6)	4(11.4)
	Using the telephone	60(83.3)	11(15.3)	1(1.4)	11(31.4)	21(60.0)	3(8.6)
	Using public transportation	59(81.9)	13(18.1)	0(0)	30(85.7)	3(8.6)	2(5.7)
	Light housework	39(54.2)	2(2.8)	2(2.8)	22(62.9)	4(11.4)	9(25.7)
	Taking care of business at a store, a hospital, and a government office				23(65.7)	3(8.6)	9(25.7)
	Food preparation				19(54.3)	8(22.9)	8(22.9)
	Heavy housework				28(80.0)	5(14.3)	2(5.7)
	Laundry				25(71.4)	5(14.3)	5(14.3)
	Responsibility for own medication				20(57.1)	7(20.0)	8(22.9)
	Handing finances				21(60.0)	5(14.3)	9(25.7)
	Grooming				9(25.7)	2(5.7)	24(68.6)
	Going out a short distance				13(37.1)	9(25.7)	13(37.1)

10-10). When analyzed according to household types, centenarians living alone were likelier to perform all items independently than centenarians living with family or in a facility(Table 10-11). However, older adults living alone needed full assistance in shopping at 66.7%, using public transportation at 66.7%, doing housework at 44.4%, and using the telephone at 11.1%. This demonstrates the importance of intervention from the local government and public space for older adults to maintain their daily lives.

Table 10-11. **Instrumental activities of daily living by household type** (From Park K *et al.* Korean centenarians: 20 years of change. Koonja Publishing Inc.; 2021, with permission)

		2001			2018								
		Age 100 and over (n=72)			Age 100 and over, living alone (n=9)			Age 100 and over, living with family (n=20)			Age 100 and over, facility resident (n=7)		
		Dependent	Slightly dependent	Independent	Dependent	Slightly dependent	Independent	Dependent	Slightly dependent	Independent	Dependent	Slightly dependent	Independent
IADL	Shopping	80.6	13.9	5.6	66.7	11.1	22.2	80.0	10.0	10.0	100	0	0
	Using the telephone	83.3	15.3	1.4	11.1	66.7	22.2	40.0	55.0	5.0	33.3	66.7	0
	Using public transportation	81.9	18.1	0	66.7	22.2	11.1	90.0	5.0	5.0	100	0	0
	Light housework	54.2	2.8	2.8	44.4	11.1	44.4	65.0	15.0	20.0	83.3	0	16.7

Summary

Foremost, centenarians' lifestyles have changed in a much healthier direction. Both 2001 and 2018 had an average of approximately 9 hours of regular sleep, and smoking and alcohol consumption were remarkably low. The range of activity has also increased. In the past, most centenarians had an activity range within their rooms. Nevertheless, in 2018, several centenarians had an activity range that reached around the village and further away. Moreover, most had under 30 min of activity duration in the past, but in the case of 2018, the number of centenarians who perform 1 to 2 hours of activities has improved immensely. This indicates that centenarians now have a higher health status than before.

Additionally, centenarians who like to socialize with others take up to half their numbers, and even those who do not have a history of good socialization but are now unable to do so due to health issues or not having suitable companions. It was established that senior citizen centers are becoming the site for these social gatherings, particularly in rural villages. This also implies that the local or national governments can help sustain these social gatherings by supporting senior citizen centers. It was shown that centenarians are maintaining and enjoying more social relationships than in the past or as expected in the present, and it is possible to interpret these social relationships makes a substantial contribution to centenarians' psychological stability and mental health. Inspection of activities of daily living and instrumental activities of daily living showed that centenarians living alone or living with family needed less help than those living in facilities, and centenarians who lived alone showed better mobility. Among instrumental activities of daily living, the item that required less total assistance compared to before was using the telephone. It is believed that this is because mobile phones are more widely distributed than before and have easier accessibility and learnability. Based on this, it can be determined that the development of science and telecommunication that helps our daily lives is also providing great help to centenarians. In contrast to 20 years ago, centenarians are leading a more active lifestyle due to advancements in medical and welfare services and technology.

References

- Park K *et al*. Korean centenarians: 20 years of change. Koonja Publishing Inc., 2021.

PART III

Chapter 11

Diets of Korean Centenarians

Clara Yongjoo Park

Introduction

For several decades, research has focused on discovering, purifying, and enriching or fortifying nutrients such as vitamins, minerals, and fatty acids. These were especially of interest due to deficiency-related health outcomes during the past centuries. Recently, with the development of the economy, agriculture, transportation, etc., food has become abundant in many developing countries. Despite the phenomenal success in medicine and the increase in life expectancy, healthy life expectancy still drags far behind life expectancy, especially in Korea [Statistics Korea 2023]. As some research on single nutrients or a combination of nutrients does not show health benefits in populations with adequate food supplies, more phytochemicals and/or the interaction between several nutrients and the food matrix must be studied. As no such 'miracle food' exists, recent research focuses on dietary patterns, more than individual nutrients or food compounds, as it encompasses all nutrients and foods and is easier to convey to the public and implement diet strategies. Regardless of the type of dietary pattern, healthier dietary patterns are associated with lower risk of chronic disease and premature death in adults. Centenarian research in Korea previously focused on dietary habits and nutrient intake. As dietary quality indexes become available for Korea, such as the Korean Healthy Eating Index (KHEI) and Nutrient Quotient (NQ), more research on diet quality of centenarians has become possible.

By comparing the dietary intakes of Korean centenarians of the early 2000's and 2020's, we can observe the changes in intake and food culture among centenarians during two decades [Lee, M-S, 2005a, 2005b; Park, S *et al.*, 2008; Kwak, CS, *et al.,* 2012; Lee, M-S, 2011]. In addition, the similarities in intake may point to some key dietary factors related to healthy longevity. Due to the limited research on the diet of Korean centenarians, we will utilize reports of 1) 54 centenarians residing in rural areas (9 counties and 2 prefectures) around Korea (mean age: 101 years) surveyed between 2001 and 2002 [Park, S *et al.*, 2008], 2) 87 adults 95 years and older living in Seoul (mean age: 96.9 years) surveyed in 2009 [Kwak, CS, *et al.*, 2012], and 3) 70 adults 95 years and older living in the Gurye, Goksung, Sunchang, and Damyang (GuGokSunDam) longevity belt (mean age 96.5 years) surveyed in 2022 [Kim, S, 2023]. Among the adults surveyed in Seoul and GuGokSunDam, centenarians made up 20% of the study population within each study. Due to the small sample size, centenarians were not separately analyzed in these studies. Therefore, due to the inability to distinguish data of centenarians and for the simplicity of writing, participants of these studies (including those 95 years of age and older) are referred to here as 'centenarians'. In addition, due to the possible differences in food culture according to region, I will also refer to some data of nonagenarians living in the GuGokSunDam longevity belt surveyed in 2003 (n=91, mean age 96.5 years) [Lee M-S, 2005a, 2005b]. The surveyed centenarians and nonagenarians were convenience samples of community-dwelling adults.

Characteristics of Korean Centenarians Associated with Diet

Stature and BMI

The height, weight, and BMI for centenarians surveyed in 2001–2002 and nonagenarians of 2003 were not reported. Centenarians of 2009 in Seoul had a mean height of 156.5 cm for men and 140.8 cm for women. Mean BMI was 21.8 and 20.9 for men and women, respectively, which did not statistically differ between sexes. For centenarians of 2022, the mean height for men and women was 148.4 cm, and the mean BMI was 19.5. Thus, although stature is similar among these centenarians, those surveyed in 2022 in GuGokSunDam were leaner than those evaluated in 2009 residing in Seoul. Underweight centenarians made up 17.2% and 35.2%, and obese participants accounted for 10.3% and 1.8% for Seoul (2009) and GuGokSunDam (2022) centenarians, respectively. The differences in BMI may be due to region and environmental differences rather than changes with time. Seoul is a large metropolitan city with good access to markets and restaurants compared to the rural areas such as GuGokSunDam.

Physical activity

Physical activity is associated with energy intake and important to enhance and maintain physical function and health in addition to its benefits for mental health. Sixty-three percent of centenarians living in rural areas in 2001–2002 reported to exercise regularly. Similarly, 73.6% of GuGokSunDam nonagenarians reported to exercise regularly. This shows that a high proportion of centenarians living in rural areas are physically active. On the other hand, among 2009 Seoul centenarians, 85.1% reported not participating in regular exercise, 40.7% reported almost no physical activity, and 50% reported less than 1 hour of physical activity per day. Living in a metropolitan city may limit the activity of centenarians. This may also explain the higher BMI of centenarians in Seoul compared to GuGokSunDam centenarians despite similar caloric intakes.

Despite the higher rate of physically active 2001–2002 centenarians, 30% were room-bound. This is almost twice the rate of Seoul centenarians (16.1%) and GuGokSunDam nonagenarians (14.3%). The sphere of activity of centenarians was not collected in 2022.

Difficulty in ingesting foods

One-third of centenarians surveyed in 2022 did not have any reported difficulties related to ingestion. Among the difficulties related to food ingestion in centenarians, difficulty in chewing or swallowing (dysphagia) was the most common symptom affecting 37%. In 2009, 68.9% of centenarians had chewing problems at least some of the time and 24.1% always had chewing difficulty. Chewing and swallowing difficulty information was not collected in the 2001–2002 centenarians. However, in nonagenarians in 2003, approximately half reported having chewing difficulty, regardless of dentures. (In these participants, most (82.4%) did not have teeth, and only 23% of men and 15% of women had dentures.) Difficulty in chewing and swallowing seems to have decreased over the decades.

Of the 2022 centenarians, constipation or diarrhea affected 28%. This is similar to the rate of centenarians 2009 who reported always having constipation (23.0%). We were unable to find data on centenarians in 2001–2002.

Dry mouth (xerostomia) was the third most common problem of 2022 centenarians, affecting 27%. No data has been collected on xerostomia in previous surveys.

Lack of appetite was present in approximately 20% of the 2022 centenarians. This is in contrast to centenarians surveyed in 2001–2002 of which over 90% reported having good appetites and enjoyed eating, and those of 2009 of which only 11.5% reported having poor appetites. Centenarians with little appetite increased 2-fold during the past 2 decades and may be a point for continuous monitoring.

Subjective and objective health

Feeling healthy may motivate older ones to keep a healthy routine and result in a virtuous cycle. In 2001–2002, 85.7% of the centenarians rated themselves to have 'good' or 'very good' health. Among nonagenarians living in GuGokSunDam (2003), 65.9% reported to have very good or good health. Similarly, 62.7% of centenarians in 2009 and 61.4% of centenarians in 2022 reported themselves to be 'healthy' or 'very healthy'. These rates of good subjective health are exceptionally higher than those of non-centenarian older adults [Han, S-H, *et al.*, 2021], even though the rate seems to gradually decrease with time. The decrease in good subjective health may be due to the increase in survival of centenarians with the help of modern medicine. In 2001–2002 only 10.7% had chronic disease; however, in 2009, 59.3% were taking some type of medication, and in 2022 only 18.6% were reported to be disease-free. In 2022, the most prevalent disease was hypertension (60.3%), followed by dementia (23.5%), osteoarthritis (17.7%), and diabetes mellitus (14.7%). The increase in medical facilities and the number of centenarians in Korea also supports that medical treatment may play a large role in centenarians' health.

Living alone

In 2022, 37.9% of the centenarians lived alone, a large increase from 2001–2002 centenarians. During the early 2000's, 94.4% of the centenarians lived with family – mostly the son and daughter-in-law or the daughter-in-law only (77.8%). Even in Seoul in 2009, only 9.2% of the centenarians were living alone. This drastic change in family structure may also affect diet, as most centenarians require help for meal preparation. While the daughter-in-law living with the centenarian was in charge of meals in the early 2000's, in 2022 the rate of sons, daughters, and daughters-in-law that purchased groceries was similar. Family members living within close proximity would stock the refrigerator and freezer with food for the centenarians during their visits. The proportion of those preparing (cooking) foods was similar among the centenarian oneself, daughter, daughter-in-law, and/or care-worker in 2022. In 2022, 59% of all participants were visited by a care worker, who may buy groceries, cook meals, or set the table for centenarians, especially those living alone. In addition, 19% of the centenarians received meal services, such as lunch boxes or banchan delivery, from social services. As the family structure of centenarians shifted towards more independent living during the decades, the meal-related responsibilities also broadened out from the daughter-in-law being solely in charge to the children of the centenarian – the son and daughter – and social welfare.

Literacy

Among the centenarians surveyed in 2022, 60.9% were unable to read. This illiteracy rate is lower than the rate of nonagenarians surveyed in 2003 with no elementary school education (81.8%) living in the same area, although some without elementary school education may still be able to read. However, the illiteracy rate is much higher than those living in Seoul surveyed in 2009 (29%; 8% in men and 37% in women). The high illiteracy rates in GuGokSunDam may be due to limited access to education in rural areas at a time in Korea when elementary school was not compulsory. In addition, those who were more educated that day may have moved to Seoul to look for work. Illiteracy may affect many aspects of life, including food purchase, understanding nutrition information, and food safety. Family members and care-givers who usually prepare the meals for centenarians were all able to read and write in 2022. Therefore, this may not have drastically affected current intake. However, this may have affected previous intake when the centenarians prepared meals for themselves.

Dietary Habits of Korean Centenarians

Regularity of meals

Most centenarians surveyed in the 2000s and 2022 ate regularly and meal sizes were consistent. Less than 6% reported having very irregular meal times, similar to the rate of centenarians who ingested very irregular meal sizes for both time points. In addition, most centenarians did not eat late at night.

Eating out (including to-go and delivery foods)

The prevalence of eating out has increased in the past decades in Korea. The mean frequency of consuming foods not prepared at home (includes dining at a restaurant, to-go/delivered foods, meals prepared and consumed at community facilities or religious organizations, etc.; excludes home-cooked meals at homes of other people) was 1.3 times/month in 2009 Seoul centenarians. For GuGokSunDam centenarians in 2022, 67% of centenarians ate out or had to-go/delivered foods less than once per month in the past year. The low rate of consuming foods prepared from places outside of a home in the GuGokSunDam residents may be due to the COVID-19 pandemic in 2020–2022, which greatly reduced community meals. In addition, Seoul is a metropolitan city with better accessibility to restaurants than rural areas such as GuGokSunDam.

Food and Nutrient Intake of Korean Centenarians

Diet quality

Diversity and balance of meals were assessed using the Koreans dietary diversity score (KDDS) and meal balance (MB) in the early 2000's. The KDDS calculates how many food groups (cereals and bread; meat, fish, eff, and legumes; dairy; vegetables and fruits; and nuts, fat, and oil) were consumed meal. A score of over 3 is thought to be a well-balanced diet. The MB is the sum of KDDS for all three-meals with a score of over 8 being preferable. Mean KDDS and MB scores of Korean centenarians in 2001–2002 were 3.52 and 8.35, respectively, indicating a relatively diverse diet. Centenarians in Seoul in 2009 had a mean score of 4.7 and 11.7 for KDDS and MB, respectively. Diet variety score (DVS) counts the number of foods ingested daily. A higher DVS indicates more variety of the diet. Centenarians in 2001–2002 and 2009 had relatively high DVS – 18.5 and 19.4, respectively. The KDDS, MB, and DVS were similar between male and female centenarians in 2009. These results show that in the early 2000's Korean centenarians had a well-balanced, diverse diet.

In 2022, diet quality was assessed using the NQ for the elderly (NQ-E). The NQ-E was developed in 2014–2015 and revised in 2021. Therefore, the NQ-E was not available in previous surveys. The NQ-E used in 2022 targets adults 65 years and older to assess nutrition status and diet quality. The NQ-E questionnaire is divided into three domains – balance, moderation, and practice – and a total score can be calculated. According to the score for each domain and total score, participants can be categorized into low, medium, and high, where a higher score indicates better nutrition status and diet quality. The mean ± standard deviation NQ-E scores of centenarians living in GuGokSunDam in 2022 were within the 'medium' category. As little research has been performed in Korean oldest-old, whether the categorization of NQ-E is applicable to the centenarians is unknown. Still, higher NQ-E relates to better diet quality. NQ-E scores were higher in females than males and in those consuming dietary supplements/functional foods. A trend for a positive relationship between NQ-E and subjective income was also observed ($p=0.06$). Unexpectedly, centenarians living alone did not have lower NQ-E than those living with others, possibly due to the visits of care workers and meal delivery from social sectors – age, living alone, and low income are the criteria to receive these services. Dietary supplement intake or nutrient intake from supplements are not included in the NQ-E questionnaire. Therefore, ingesting dietary supplements/functional foods seems to indicate the family support and motivation of the centenarian to stay in good health, and is reflected in food intake and thus a higher NQ. Thus, the diet quality of current Korean centenarians is modest and may differ by sex, and familial and social support.

Some studies indicate that centenarians' dietary patterns or quality are 'healthier' compared to younger generations – however, whether this is a longevity-related pattern or a generation and cultural difference is unclear. For instance, centenarians of Georgia, USA consumed more whole milk than their counter parts. In Japanese centenarians, those who consumed a dietary pattern preferring dairy had a higher survival rate compared to those preferring beverages [Shimizu, K, *et al.*, 2003]. Milk may be associated with longevity due to its protein and calcium content. However, centenarians of Korea ingest little dairy, as will be discussed below. Likewise, foods known as 'healthy' and expected to be consumed more by centenarians are not always ingested more than others. For instance, centenarians of Japan and Georgia, USA both consume less fish than their counter parts [Hausman, DB, *et al.*, 2011]. In addition, from several studies, centenarians did not consistently consume more vegetables than their younger counterparts. As most studies are cross-sectional, more long-term follow-up studies are required to assess the effect of dietary patterns on the longevity of centenarians.

Food groups

Investigating food intake in centenarians is exceptionally difficult. Remembering the variety and amount of one's intake requires much effort and may not be reliable, regardless of age [Willett, W, 2012]. Reports can vary by season or day of the week. This may be even more so in centenarians as their memory deteriorates with age, and they are usually not involved in the preparation of meals. In addition, hearing loss and low rate of literacy of Korean centenarians is a large barrier to communication. We surveyed centenarians and care-givers, including children or grandchildren and social workers that cared for their meals, to assess food and nutrition intake. In the early 2000's food intake was assessed by interviews, surveillance of foods in centenarians' refrigerators, and asking the one responsible for the centenarians' meals to replicate the previous meal ingested [Lee, M-S, 2005b]. However, this demands enormous amounts of time and energy and has not been validated. In 2022, with the development and wide use of electronic devices, we were able to record meals to assess food intake less intrusively and more accurately, as reliance on memory was unnecessary. One hundred twenty-eight videos of meals from 19 centenarians were analyzed by trained research staff to analyze the amount of foods and nutrients consumed. The characteristics (age, distribution of sex, subjective income, living alone, etc) of centenarians that agreed to record meals and those that did not did not differ.

1) Grains

Rice is the main cereal for Koreans. Therefore, cereals (mostly rice) make up a large portion of daily intake. Despite the lower energy intake, nonagenarians and centenarians ingested more rice and approximately two times more potatoes compared to nationally representative intakes of adults 65 years and older. One may think that this may be due to the surveys being implemented in a rural area in the summer – a season when potatoes are harvested. However, similar amounts were consumed in centenarians Seoul, a large metropolitan city, in 2009 as well. Potatoes may be a preferred starchy food by centenarians as they are easier to ingest when having difficulty chewing.

No data was reported on whole grains and multi-grains in 2001−2002 or 2009 centenarians. In nonagenarians of 2003, most consumed white rice rather than brown rice or mixed grain. However, in 2022, 43% of the centenarians consumed whole grains or multigrains twice or more times a day.

2) Meat, fish, eggs, and legumes

Centenarians in 2001−2002 consumed meat, fish, eggs, and soybean products 11 times per week (meat and fish: 4 times a week; eggs: 2.3 times per week; soybean products: 4.7 times per week), which is similar to nonagenarians in 2003. The amount of meat, fish, eggs, and legumes (in g) is much higher in centenarians in Seoul (2009) than nonagenarians in 2003. Seoul centenarians consumed 2∼4 fold more meat, fish and legumes than GuGokSunDam nonagenarians. For instance, men consumed 152.7 g/d and 43.9 g/d and women ingested 76.4 mg/d and 39.3 mg/d of meat in Seoul centenarians and GuGokSunDam nonagenarians, respectively. Men consumed similar amounts of eggs (14.1 vs. 9.5 g/d for Seoul and GuGokSunDam, respectively), but women residing in Seoul ingested more eggs than those in GuGokSunDam (28.1 vs. 8.0 g/d). Centenarians of Seoul also consumed more meat, eggs, and legumes than the nationally representative intakes of Koreans 65 years and older. These observations indicate that intakes of protein foods may drastically differ by region.

3) Vegetables and seaweeds

Vegetable intake was not reported in 2001−2002 centenarians. In nonagenarians of 2003, mean daily vegetable intakes were 276.6 g (including 145.6 g of kimchi) for men and 177.7 g (including 57.6 g of kimchi) for women. This seems lower than the intakes of Seoul centenarians in 2009, which reached a mean of 357.4 and 339.5 g/d for men and women, respectively.

In 2001−2002 centenarians, seaweeds were consumed 4.4 times per week. Nonagenarians of 2003 consumed seaweed 2.9

times per day and amounted to 2.5 g in men and 2.9 g in women per day. Seoul centenarian men consumed less (0.7 g/d) and women consumed more (3.6 g/d) than nonagenarians of GuGokSunDam.

4) Fruit and dairy

Nonagenarians residing in GuGokSunDam consumed very little fruits (mean: 53 g [approximately one-third of a serving] per day), despite their high preference for fruits and despite it being summer in a rural area. Dairy consumption was also very low – mean: 4.1 g/d for men and 29.4 g/d for women. For reference, one cup of milk is 200−250 g. Thus, hardly any milk or dairy was consumed in this population, – On the other hand, centenarians in 2009 living in Seoul consumed more fruit and dairy compared to those in GuGokSunDam, regardless of year. Mean daily fruit intake was more than 4-fold that of GuGokSunDam nonagenarians (~230 g). Mean dairy intake reached 152.2 g/d. The difference between GuGokSunDam and Seoul centenarians may be due to income and culture. Fruit is expensive in Korea and fresh fruit cannot be stored for a long time. In addition, Koreans typically do not consume much dried or canned fruits. GuGokSunDam is located in mountainous areas, and thus, less fruit may be available even in summer. We did not observe many fruit trees in the gardens of the homes of centenarians. Similarly, dairy is relatively expensive and has a short storage life. In addition, dairy is not included in the traditional Korean diet and many older ones may have lactose intolerance. Therefore, centenarians in rural areas may not be accustomed to dairy and may not be able to afford dairy and fruit as much as those living in metropolitan areas. These results indicate that consumption of fruit and dairy may differ between centenarians living in rural areas and those living in Seoul metropolitan city.

5) Oils and sweets

Fat and oil consumption was greater in Seoul centenarians compared to nonagenarians in GuGokSunDam. No data is available for 2001–2002 and 2022 centenarians. Nonagenarians of GuGokSunDam in 2003 consumed 4.8 g/d mostly as oil. Seoul centenarians ingested a mean of 16.1 g/d, approximately 3-fold more than GuGokSunDam participants. Nuts were not reported separately in previous studies; however, intakes of nuts seem to be close to zero. Nuts are not part of the traditional diet of Koreans, are expensive (except for peanuts), have short storage life due to the high-fat content, and are difficult to chew for most centenarians. Nut butters and powders are not commonly consumed in Korea, especially for the older population.

Despite the low energy intake of nonagenarians compared to younger generations, nonagenarians ingested approximately two times more sugary foods compared to nationally representative intakes of adults 65 years and older. Seoul-residing centenarians ingested similar amounts. Similarly, 2022 centenarians reported to commonly enjoy instant coffee and candy. This may be because the survey is implemented in the summer when ice cream and cold, sugary drinks are preferred. In addition, some centenarians frequently consumed candy throughout the day to prevent the discomfort of dry mouth.

Nutrient intake

In the below section, we refer to the Dietary Reference Intakes for Koreans (KDRIs) in order to help understand the context of nutrient intake. However, as the physiology of centenarians may differ and dietary guidelines are not available specifically for centenarians, these do not accurately reflect adequacy or deficiency. In addition, caution is needed when interpreting changes in nutrient intakes. Due to the change in the method of survey between years (simulated previous meal vs. video recording), the differences in analyzed nutrient values may represent measurement error rather than actual difference in intake. Therefore, when discussing changes here, I focus on values with large differences unlikely to be due to systematic error.

1) **Energy and macronutrients**

The energy intake of centenarians has been reported to be lower than younger generations in many studies throughout the world [Hausman, DB, *et al.*, 2011]. This was also consistently observed in Korean centenarians throughout the decades. Centenarians of 2001−2002. 2009, and 2022 ingested approximately 1300 kcal/d. Centenarians were consuming approximately 75% of the recommended dietary allowances (RDA) or estimated energy requirements for Koreans 75 years and older (per sex). Carbohydrate intakes decreased, fat intake increased while protein intakes were similar throughout the years; This is similar to the changes in the intakes of non-centenarian Korean adults [Oh, SW, 2022].

2) **Vitamins**

Vitamin A and vitamin C intakes decreased by approximately 50% during the two decades. On the contrary, vitamin B_1 and B_6, folate, and vitamin E intakes increased over two-fold during the past two decades. Still, approximately 30−70% of the surveyed centenarians did not meet the Recommended Nutrient I ntakes (RNI).

3) **Minerals**

Dietary calcium intake is consistently low among centenarians, similar to the general adult population. Mean calcium from diet was approximately 376.2 mg/d in 2001−2002. The mean intakes of 2022 also fall far below the recommended intakes for older Koreans (40∼50% of the RDA or RNI). This may be due to the low intake of dairy. Older adults are reported to have a high intake of total calcium, due to the use of dietary supplements. However, only a few centenarians that we surveyed in 2022 were taking dietary supplements that included calcium. On the other hand, phosphorus intakes were relatively unchanged (~620 mg/d) throughout the decades. The mean intakes met approximately 90% of the RNI and were lower than the general population (>1000 mg/d for adults 19–64 years, 878.6 mg/d for adults ≥ 65 years [KHIDI 2020]). Interestingly, only 10.3% of these centenarians had osteoporosis despite the low calcium intake.

By 2022, mean zinc intakes met the RNI; however, the intakes may have been skewed as half the population did not meet the RNI.

Despite intakes of many nutrients not meeting the recommendations for older adults, the mean iron intake of centenarians was relatively high, with over 70% meeting the recommended intakes. Iron intakes increased, while potassium tended to decrease during the decades and remained below the mean intake of adults 65 years and older. Sodium intake decreased during the decades but was consistently high and is far beyond the Upper Level for sodium (2000 mg/d). The intakes are similar to the general population and reflect the decrease in sodium intake of Korean adults throughout the years [Park, CY *et al.*, 2020]. However, although most nutrient intakes of centenarians are lower than younger generations, the 2022 centenarians' intake for sodium is *higher* than the mean for adults 65 years and older in 2020 [KHIDI, 2020].

4) Fiber

Fiber intake was 5.2 g/d in 2002–2002 centenarians. This increased nearly 4-fold in 2022 centenarians. This shows that the decrease in vitamins may not be due to a decrease in vegetable intake. It is possible that the higher proportion of centenarians consuming whole grain/mixed grain in 2022 affected the mean fiber intake.

Supplements

In the early 2000's, only a few centenarians were taking dietary supplements. Among the 2001–2002 centenarians in Korea, only 16.7% were consuming supplements. Similarly, only 12.6% of Seoul centenarians were taking dietary supplements or functional foods in 2009. However, we found in 2022 that over half of the centenarians in GuGokSunDam were taking dietary supplements/functional foods/herbal medicines. This trend reflects the increase in use of dietary supplements and functional foods but shows a delayed but rapid increase in the oldest-old. The dietary supplements and functional foods commonly consumed included multi-vitamins, multi-minerals, probiotics (and prebiotics), protein powder, traditional Korean herbal medicine, etc. These were provided mainly by children of the centenarian and some from local public health centers.

Summary

Our research shows that the close environment – such as family support and living conditions, social benefits, etc. – has changed throughout the decades. Recently, more family members than just the daughter-in-law prepared meals for the centenarian. Centenarians that felt 'healthy' or 'very heathy' decreased during the past decades but were still much higher than non-centenarians. The decrease may be due to the actual decrease in centenarians without a medical diagnosis.

Interestingly, despite the changes in the local environment that may affect food intake, energy, food, and nutrient intake have not changed much over the past two decades. Centenarians consume less energy and nutrients than younger generations. The low intake of fruit, dairy, and nuts may by typical to Korean traditional diets, and owing to the low accessibility (due to high cost and low shelf life) and difficulty in mastication and digestion of these foods. The changes in the diet of centenarians mostly reflect changes in the Korean population and do not seem to be specific to centenarians.

However, we do see that regional differences may exist when comparing centenarians residing in Seoul with those residing in rural areas. Seoul centenarians tend to be less physically active and consume more fat/oil, dairy, and fruit. However, the intakes of dairy and fruit are still very low. The difference in intakes between centenarians residing in Seoul versus rural areas may be due to the higher income level of centenarians and/or their care givers, better accessibility to fresh fruit and dairy, and less access to parks or places to physical activity of the former.

As the 2022 research on diet was performed on centenarians of Jeollado province, the results may also include dietary habits and family customs of Jeollado province, not specifically those of centenarians. However, as no research on centenarians has been completed recently in other regions in Korea, comparing the intakes of our participants with nationally representative intakes of older adults, such as utilizing the Korea National Health and Nutrition Examination Survey (KNHANES), may be helpful. KNHANES includes geographic regions, making it also possible to rule out regional traits. In addition, by prospectively assessing the intakes of older adults in Korea, we may discover some distinctions of Korean centenarians' diet.

To conclude, centenarians of the past two decades have changed little in their dietary habits – most of the changes reflecting changes in the Korean diet in general. Further research is required to assess centenarians residing in various regions of Korea. In addition, more in-depth investigation is necessary to understand the specifics of centenarians' dietary habits and nutrition status.

References

- Han S-H, Kang JK, Hong J-S. A Study of Factors Related to the Subjective Health Status of Elderly Population in Korea. Health Policy and Management 2021;56-64.
- Hausman DB, Fischer JG, Johnson MA. Nutrition in centenarians. Maturitas 2011;68(3):203-209.
- KHIDI. National Nutrition Statistics. Nutrient intakes 2020 [cited Sept 11, 2023; Available from: https://www.khidi.or.kr/kps/dhraStat/result5?menuId=MENU01656&gubun=age1&year=2020.
- Kim S, Dietary habits and nutritional intake of adults 95 years and older living in the Gugoksundam longevity belt, Department of Food and Nutrition, Chonnam National University Graduate School, 2023.
- Kwak CS, Cho JH, Yon M, Park SC. Anthropometric index, dietary habits and nutrient intake of the oldest-old population aged 95 and over living in Seoul. Korean Journal of Community Nutrition 2012;17(5):603-622.
- Lee M-S. The dietary habits of the nonagenarian population in longevity belt in Korea. Korean Journal of Community Nutrition 2005a;513-524.
- Lee M-S. Nutritional status of the nonagenarian population in longevity belt in Korea. Korean Journal of Community Nutrition 2005b;290-302.
- Lee M-S. Dietary habits and nutritional characteristics of Korean centenarians. Food Industry And Nutrition 2011;16(2):27-33.
- Oh SW. Current status of nutrient intake in Korea; focused on macro-nutrients. J Korean Med Assoc 2022;65(12):801-809.
- Park CY, Jo G, Lee J, Singh GM, Lee J-T, Shin M-J. Association between dietary sodium intake and disease burden and mortality in Koreans between 1998 and 2016: The Korea National Health and Nutrition Examination Survey. Nutrition Research and Practice 2020;14(5):501-518.
- Park SC, Lee MS, Kwon IS, Kwak CS, Yeo EJ. Environment and gender influences on the nutritional and health status of Korean centenarians. Asian J Gerontol Geriatr 2008;3(2):75-83.

- Shimizu K, Takeda S, Noji H, Hirose N, Ebihara Y, Arai Y, Hamamatsu M, Nakazawa S, Gondo Y, Konishi K. Dietary Patterns and Further Survival in Japanese Centenarians. Journal of Nutritional Science and Vitaminology 2003;49(2):133-138.
- Statistics Korea, Life Expectancy at Birth (0 years) and Expected Life Span Excluding Morbidity (Healthy Life Expectancy). [Accessed September 11, 2023]; Available from: https://www.index.go.kr/unity/potal/main/EachDtlPageDetail.do?idx_cd=2758.
- Willett W. Nutritional Epidemiology. Oxford University Press, 2012.

Chapter 12

The Immunity of Centenarians

the Secret to Maintaining a Healthy Life and Surviving COVID-19

Kyung A Cho

As we age, our immune system undergoes a gradual decline in function, which makes us more vulnerable to infections, cancers, and other diseases. This phenomenon is called immunosenescence, and various changes in the composition, distribution, and activity of immune cells and molecules characterize it. One of the hallmarks of immunosenescence is inflammaging, a low-grade chronic inflammation that persists throughout life and contributes to age-related tissue damage and dysfunction(Figure 12-1). Inflammaging is thought to be caused by multiple factors, such as cell senescence, oxidative stress, mitochondrial dysfunction, and dysregulated cytokine signaling. These factors interact, and genetic and environmental factors shape the trajectory of immunosenescence and its consequences for health and longevity. For example, inflammaging has been linked to age-related conditions like Alzheimer's disease, cardiovascular disease, and frailty, as well as to mortality and disability. Investigators at the Stanford University School of Medicine and the Buck Institute for Research on Aging have built an inflammatory-aging clock

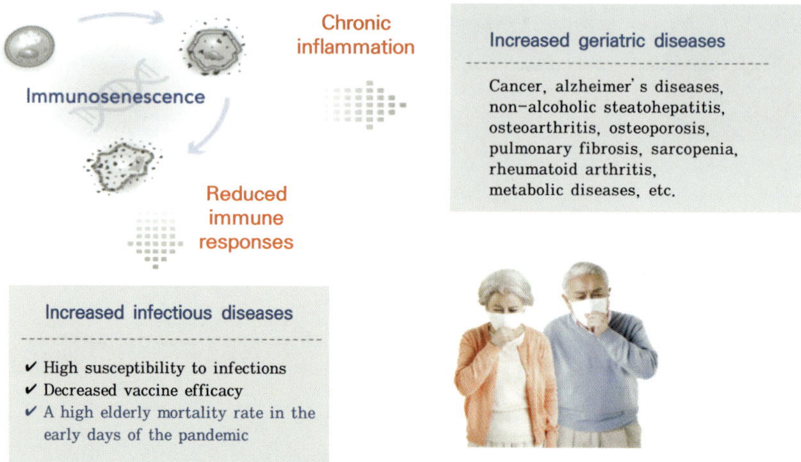

Figure 12-1. The onset of geriatric diseases due to immunosenescence

that's more accurate than the number of candles on your birthday cake in predicting how strong your immune system is, how soon you will become frail or whether you have unseen cardiovascular problems that could become clinical headaches a few years down the road. "Every year, the calendar tells us we are a year older," said Dr. David Furman, the study's senior author. "But not all humans age biologically at the same rate. You see this in the clinic – some older people are extremely disease-prone, while others are the picture of health." Interestingly, Centenarians show remarkable exceptions to the typical pattern of immunosenescence and inflammaging. Recent studies have shown that centenarians have a distinct profile of immune cells and molecules, characterized by lower levels of pro-inflammatory cytokines and higher levels of anti-inflammatory cytokines and a better balance between innate and adaptive immunity. In addition, centenarians seem to have a higher capacity for immunoregulation, which allows them to dampen excessive immune responses and prevent autoimmune diseases.

The immune system of centenarians has attracted increasing attention from researchers who seek to understand the secrets of healthy aging and longevity. By studying the genetics, epigenetics, and environmental factors that shape the immune system of centenarians, scientists hope to identify new targets for interventions that can delay or prevent age-related diseases and disabilities. Moreover, the immune system of centenarians may provide clues to the evolution and adaptation of human immunity over time and across populations. Centenarians possess the secrets to maintaining a healthy life for an extended period; one of these secrets is a robust immune system. This fact became apparent during the early days of the COVID-19 pandemic, when the world was under lockdown, and the mortality rate among older people rapidly increased. However, centenarians showed a relatively low mortality rate and

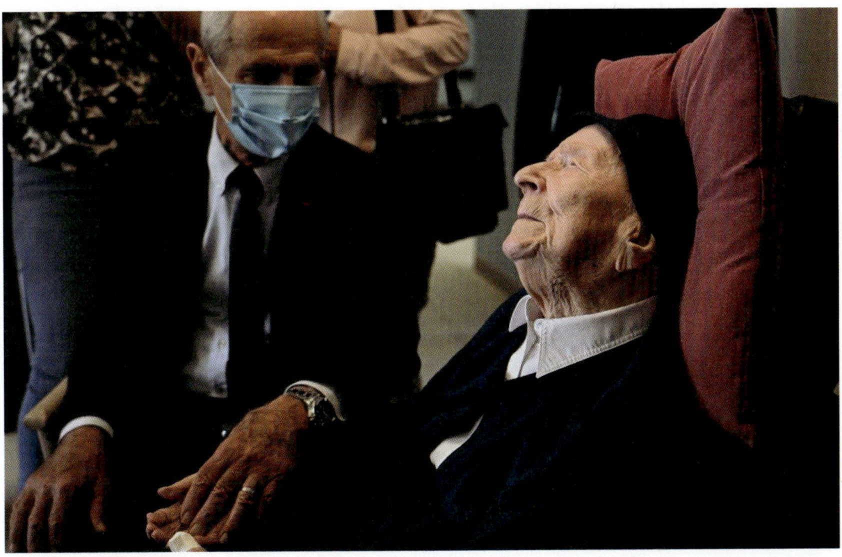

Figure 12-2. Recovered from COVID-19, Sister Lucile Randon and Director Fauci @ CNN April 27, 2022

healthy recovery after infection, drawing attention to their immunity. For example, at 117, Sister Lucile Randon from France recovered from COVID-19 and inspired people worldwide(Figure 12-2).

Similarly, from the Ivanovo region in western Russia, news broke out about a 101-year-old grandmother who was in critical condition due to COVID-19 but eventually recovered her health and was discharged, which made the world admire the resilience of centenarians. In the United States, news reports highlighted the high survival rate among centenarians, with all but three of the 60 centenarians recovering healthily from the virus. Professor Sang Chul Park, who led a study on centenarians in South Korea, posited that centenarians' significantly lower fasting blood sugar and glycated hemoglobin might contribute to their superior health and longevity. His studies showed that compared to the general population, centenarians had a much lower prevalence of hypertension and diabetes. Japanese centenarian data supported this, demonstrating reduced rates of these conditions as individuals aged. This low incidence of baseline diseases, lifestyle habits, and robust immune systems may contribute to their resistance to infectious diseases like COVID-19. Although some argue that centenarians may have been better protected than the general elderly population, subsequent research has shown that the unique immune system of centenarians can contribute to their high survival rate. Various research analyzed the importance of immune responses in maintaining the health of centenarians by studying their unique immune responses. They found that centenarians have a distinct profile of immune cells and molecules, characterized by lower levels of pro-inflammatory cytokines and higher levels of anti-inflammatory cytokines, as well as a better balance between innate and adaptive immunity. Additionally, centenarians seem to have a higher capacity for immunoregulation, which allows them to dampen excessive immune responses and prevent autoimmune diseases [Moskalev A, *et al.*, 2020].

In this chapter, we will provide a comprehensive overview of the unique immune system of centenarians that enables them to resist diseases and maintain their health, covering multiple perspectives. Additionally, we will explore the relationship between this unique immune system and health maintenance in centenarians. The Unique Immunity of Centenarians possesses astonishing vitality. One of the secrets to their healthy lives is their powerful immune system, which helps them resist age-related diseases and maintain a healthy lifestyle.

The Immune System of Centenarians has Some Unique Features

Distinctive cell types: Ratio of T cells and B cells

In April 2023, as a research result was reported, the media focused on "Robust Immunity May Be Key to Centenarian's Longevity" as a headline. The research has found that the blood of centenarians contains unique immune cell types compared to the average population. This study observed individual immune responses in populations aged 100 or older. The researchers analyzed the types and quantities of immune cells by collecting blood samples from healthy people aged 100 or older, healthy populations aged 80 or older, and healthy populations in their 20s. As a result, the 100+ age group showed a higher number of B cells and fewer T cells than the other two groups. In addition, these immune responses were robust in the ability to produce antibodies, and the ability to produce antibodies against specific bacteria and viruses was exceptionally high. The researchers speculate that these immune responses with higher B cell and lower T cell levels may play an essential role in maintaining the health of the 100+ age group. These results may help understand age-related changes in the immune system and may help develop ways to prevent or treat these changes [Karagiannis TT, *et al.*, 2023].

These cell types help them combat age-related diseases such as infections and inflammation. Centenarians have an enhanced quantity and quality of highly specialized immune cells, explicitly circulating T-cells and B-cells. T-cells recognize and eliminate infected cells, while B-cells produce antibodies that attack foreign invaders. The T-cells and B-cells of centenarians possess a higher antigen recognition ability and quicker response time, allowing them to effectively combat infections and age-related diseases.

Changes in the immune system: low inflammation

One of the hallmarks of immunosenescence is inflammaging, a low-grade chronic inflammation that persists throughout life and contributes to age-related tissue damage and dysfunction [Chambers and Akbar. 2020; Chung HY, *et al.*, 2009]. However, centenarians seem to possess a unique immune system more effective at suppressing age-related inflammation and reducing the risk of related diseases. As individuals age, there's a discernible rise in proinflammatory cytokines and a decline in anti-inflammatory cytokines in their plasma. Notably, in centenarians, inflammatory and anti-inflammatory markers, such as CRP, IL-12, TNF-α, IFN-γ, IL-6, and IL-10, are even more pronounced than in other older adults. Yet, for cytokines like IL-17A, IL-1β, IL-23, and TGF-β, the levels in centenarians mirror those of younger individuals. Within this context, Th17 cells, specialized subsets of CD4+ T cells that often mediate proinflammatory responses, especially in autoimmune conditions, appear less inclined to produce such responses in centenarians. On the other hand, Treg cells, which play a crucial role in maintaining immune balance by suppressing excessive immune activities, seem to lean more towards anti-inflammatory cytokine production, even though they are somewhat diminished in centenarians. From these insights, it's inferred that centenarians might combat the persistent low-grade inflammation seen with aging, known as inflammaging, by delicately balancing the Th17 and Treg cell dynamics and guiding them towards anti-inflammatory secretion patterns. Such observations grant us a fresh viewpoint on the mechanisms behind successful aging [Zhou L, *et al.*, 2022]. This finding is significant because age-related inflammation has been linked to various diseases, including Alzheimer's disease, cardiovascular disease, and frailty, as well as to mortality and disability. By having a lower inflammation level, centenarians are less likely to develop these age-related diseases, which contribute to a decline in quality of life and an increased risk of death. The reason behind the lower inflammation level of centenarians has yet to be fully understood, but several factors have been proposed. One possible factor is the presence of genetic variants that affect the immune response and regulate inflammation. For example, a study of Italian centenarians found a higher frequency of variants in the CDKN2A/B gene cluster, which regulates cell senescence and inflammation [Grinovich A, *et al.*, 2021]. Another possible factor is a history of exposure to various infections and stressors, which may have trained the immune system to be more resilient and adaptive. In addition to having a lower inflammation level, centenarians also exhibit a better balance between innate and adaptive immunity, which are two arms of the immune system that work together to defend against pathogens and tumors. Innate immunity is the first line of defense and includes cells such as natural killer cells and macrophages, which can recognize and eliminate pathogens without prior exposure. Adaptive immunity is the second line of defense and includes T cells and B cells, which can mount a specific response to a particular pathogen or tumor. Centenarians have a more balanced and coordinated innate-adaptive immune system, which allows them to respond effectively to different challenges while avoiding excessive inflammation or autoimmunity. For example, an epigenetic study on Japanese centenarians, while their DNA showed younger signs in areas linked to cancer and mental health, it was notably older in genes associated with TGF-β signaling. This signaling is crucial for anti-inflammatory responses and is key to healthy aging [Komaki S, *et al.*, 2023].

Microbiome

The human microbiome, particularly the gut microbiome, has emerged as a focal point in the exploration of healthy aging and longevity. This complex ecosystem of bacteria, fungi, and other microorganisms plays a pivotal role in our health, influencing everything from metabolism and immunity to neurological activity and bone density. Research indicates that the equilibrium between humans and their resident microbes is integral for mitigating age-related inflammatory processes, maintaining the intestinal barrier, and even preventing declines in bone and cognitive health.

To further elucidate this, a groundbreaking study delved into the phylogenetic microbiota analysis of semi-supercentenarians (those aged 105-109), comparing them to adults, the elderly, and centenarians

[Biagi, *et al.,* 2016]. This revealed a core set of frequently occurring, symbiotic bacterial taxa, with their abundance diminishing as age progresses. However, the intricacies of aging bring forth an increased abundance of subdominant species and a rearrangement of their co-occurrence networks. Notably, despite the changes accommodating opportunistic bacteria, certain bacterial groups, such as Akkermansia, Bifidobacterium, and Christensenellaceae, might play a pivotal role in promoting health during aging. Complementing this, another recent research led by Honda delved deeper into the gut microbiome's role in longevity [Sato Y, *et al.*, 2021]. The gut microbiome is integral to various bodily functions, from digestion and bone density to neuronal activity and immunity. Honda's research posits that the gut microbiota might be a vital external factor in preventing age-related diseases in long-living individuals. To probe this, Honda's team analyzed fecal samples from 160 Japanese centenarians, comparing them to samples from older adults around the age of 85 and younger individuals approximately 30 years old. Their findings were revelatory, showing that the microbiomes of centenarians were distinct, especially with a heightened abundance of genes inducible by bile acid. One such bile acid, isoallolithocholic acid (isoalloLCA), which plays a crucial role in metabolic and immune responses of the host, was found enriched in centenarian samples. These findings hint at the potential role of isoalloLCA-producing bacteria in promoting longevity by warding off certain pathogens and maintaining gut balance. While the direct cause-effect relationship is still under exploration, such findings spotlight the significance of beneficial bacteria in the quest for healthy aging. Honda's focus now shifts to the potential therapeutic applications of these findings, especially against infections like C. difficile. Both these studies collectively pave the way for future endeavors aiming to decode the microbiome's role in human longevity and strategize interventions for fostering healthy aging.

The Inheritance of longevity: exploring the immune systems of centenarian offspring

Interestingly, centenarians may be enriched for genes contributing to their longevity, some of which may affect immune function. From a comparative study between Sicilian centenarian offspring and age-matched controls, centenarian offspring could be inherited these genes and exhibit increased resistance to immunosenescence, the age-related decline in immune function [Rubino G, *et al.,* 2019]. The study focused on the adaptive T-cell arm of the immune system, particularly the numbers and proportions of CD4(+) and CD8(+) early- and late-differentiated T cells, as well as potentially senescent CD8(+) T cells. The results indicated that centenarian offspring displayed significant differences in these cell populations compared to the control group. Specifically, the adaptive T-cell arm of the immune system appeared more "youthful" in centenarian offspring, with differences in the numbers and proportions of both CD4(+) and CD8(+) early- and late-differentiated T cells. Additionally, potentially senescent CD8(+) T cells were found in lower numbers among centenarian offspring than in the control group. These findings suggest that centenarian offspring may have a superior ability to mount effective responses against newly encountered antigens, leading to better protection against infection and ultimately contributing to their potential longevity. Furthermore, studying centenarian offspring reveal that several B cell immune parameters are better preserved than in age-matched controls, and together with their genetic background, could contribute to their healthier aging [Bulati M, *et al.*, 2011; Colonna-Romano G, *et al.*, 2010]. The study's findings provide valuable insights into the genetic factors that may contribute to the impressive longevity of centenarians and their offspring. Furthermore, by understanding the role of immune function in the inheritance of longevity, researchers can better comprehend the complex interplay between genetics and aging. Moreover, these findings could inform future research to improve immune function and enhance overall human longevity. In conclusion, the study of centenarian offspring and their more "youthful" immune systems offers a promising avenue for understanding the inheritance of longevity and the role of immune function in this process.

Autoimmune disease onset suppression

In today's medical landscape, autoimmune diseases have risen to prominence as a leading health concern. They stand not only as one of the top ten causes of mortality for women but also as the second most prevalent cause of chronic illness in the United States. Furthermore, their presence acts as a predisposing factor to other serious conditions, such as cardiovascular diseases and cancer. Notably, patients suffering from certain autoimmune diseases often experience a truncated lifespan, becoming a tangible representation of accelerated immunosenescence. In contrast to this somber picture, centenarians paint a hopeful portrait of successful aging. These remarkable individuals consistently exhibit a robust and well-preserved immune system, characterized by lower levels of autoantibodies, a feature often associated with reduced vulnerability to autoimmune disorders. The study at hand embarked on an ambitious journey to explore the interplay between longevity and the prevalence of certain autoimmune and allergic diseases across 29 developed nations under the Organisation for Economic Co-operation and Development (OECD) [Lens-Pechakova LS, *et al.*, 2016]. The objective was multifaceted: to discern clear patterns in aging data, identify common determinants, and uncover novel factors contributing to healthy aging and longevity. The study reported here focused on clarifying the connection between longevity and some autoimmune and allergic diseases in 29 developed Organization for Economic Co-operation and Development (OECD) countries because multidisciplinary analyses of the accelerated or delayed aging data could show a distinct relationship pattern help to identify common factors and determine new essential factors that contribute to longevity and healthy aging. Through meticulous analyses, encompassing mortality rates data of diseases like multiple sclerosis (MS), rheumatoid arthritis (RA), and asthma, as well as the incidence rates of type 1 diabetes (T1D), striking findings emerged. When juxtaposed with centenarian rates and life expectancy data, an inverse linear correlation surfaced. To put it plainly, nations recording higher mortality rates from the aforementioned diseases, coupled with increased T1D incidences in children, consistently reported lower centenarian rates and reduced life expectancies. This groundbreaking discovery, the first of its kind, suggests a probable existence of shared mechanistic pathways. These pathways seem to influence both autoimmune diseases and longevity processes, albeit in opposing directions.

Why do Centenarians have Enhanced Immune Function and Recovery Ability?

Various possibilities have been suggested so far, such as genetics, lifestyle habits, and environmental factors all influencing the immune system of centenarians.

1) Genetics: It is known that genetic mutations related to the immune ability of centenarians play a role. Specific genetic

mutations found among older adults are estimated to help their immune system function more effectively. In addition, these genetic mutations increase resistance to infection, inflammation, cancer, and other diseases, contributing to maintaining a healthy state.

2) Lifestyle habits: Healthy lifestyle habits also positively impact the immune system of centenarians. Balanced diets, appropriate exercise, rest, and stress management are critical in enhancing immune system function. Centenarians can strengthen their immune systems by continuously practicing these healthy lifestyle habits.

3) Environmental factors: Centenarians' living environments also affect their health. Clean air and water, nutrient-rich foods, social support, and medical infrastructure in the area where centenarians reside all consent and strengthen their immune systems.

4) Microbiome: Recent studies have shown that the balance of microorganisms in the intestines of centenarians can positively impact their immune system. Intestinal organisms play an essential role in the body's immune response, and it is known that the microbiome of centenarians has a technical characteristic compared to other age groups. These characteristics can help strengthen the immune system of centenarians and maintain a healthy state.

5) Delay of Immune Senescence: Centenarians can delay immune senescence associated with impaired immune cell function. This means that the immune system of centenarians can be activated and processed for a more extended period. Delaying immune senescence increases resistance to infection, cancer, and other diseases and helps maintain a healthy life.

6) The adaptability of the Immune System: Centenarians' immune systems have adaptability over time. This allows them to cope

with the changes that occur during the aging process and maintain immune system function. This adaptability is vital in enhancing centenarians' immune activity and recovery ability.

Therefore, centenarians commonly have high immune activation and recovery ability for the above reasons. These abilities help them maintain a healthy state and prevent aging-related diseases.

Exploring Methods to Boost Immunosenescence

In our quest to emulate the 'super immunity' observed in centenarians, identifying targets that induce similar immune responses is crucial. While the initial stages of research hint at promising results, the journey to uncovering immune inducers analogous to the immunity exhibited by centenarians is still nascent, and considerable time and effort are required.

Geroprotectors

Interestingly, recent developments in the field of aging have seen the advent of various geroprotectors. These are substances designed to delay aging by targeting the principal mechanisms that change with aging.

A growing body of research and experimentation is being undertaken with the anticipation that these geroprotectors could potentially boost immunosenescence, thereby improving immune aging. Several geroprotectors currently under development or study include rapalogs, metformin, young blood factors, senolytics, NAD+ boosters, aspirin, and stem and immune cell repletion. These substances, operating through distinct mechanisms, are known to have effects in anti-aging and functional improvement. The recent global pandemic has underscored the urgent need for such developments. The pandemic has particularly highlighted the vulnerability of the elderly population, who have experienced higher fatality rates, leading to widespread devastation. In preparation for potential future pandemics, interest in developing immune boosters capable of enhancing aging immunity is deepening. Particular attention is being paid to proving the immunosenescence-boosting effects of existing anti-aging drugs [Zhavoronkov A. 2020]. For instance, one of the rapalogs, rapamycin, has already been clinically tested on a large scale as a vaccine adjuvant for the elderly, and some of its effects have been validated. However, the search for more specific immune boosters to effectively improve elderly immunity against pandemics or numerous infectious diseases remains imperative. Identifying and developing these boosters will be vital in fortifying our defense against infectious diseases, particularly in the aging population, and mitigating the impact of future health crises.

TLR5 as a potent target for vaccine adjuvant for the elderly

The Role of TLR5 in Enhancing Immunosenescence and its Potential as an Immunobooster Toll-like receptor 5 (TLR5) stands out as a crucial component in the immune system, particularly in the realm of immunosenescence. This protein, part of the Toll-like receptors (TLRs) family, is vital for recognizing foreign substances and activating the immune response leading to have garnered significant attention as targets for vaccine adjuvants. Unlike most TLRs, which tend to see a decline in expression or function in the context of aging immunity, TLR5 exhibits enduring activity and remains well-preserved in the immune system of the elderly. This distinctive characteristic has spurred a surge in interest in its potential as a target for developing immunoboosters aimed at enhancing aging-related immunity. By specifically recognizing bacterial flagellin, a component of the flagellum in motile bacteria, TLR5 plays an indispensable role in defending against bacterial infections. The preservation of TLR5 function in the elderly underscores its significance and opens up opportunities for harnessing its capabilities to mitigate the impacts of infectious diseases, especially in an aging population. The development of TLR5-targeted immunoboosters could have profound implications, offering a valuable avenue for enhancing the health and vitality of older individuals. As we face the ongoing challenges of emerging and re-emerging infectious threats, such innovations are pivotal in providing better protection and improving the overall well-being of the elderly.

In 2015, a study led by Prof. Kyung A Cho's research team revealed that the expression of TLR5 is well-maintained in aging immune cells and does not decrease [Lim JS, *et al.*, 2015]. The team observed the efficacy of TLR5 as an adjuvant for a pneumonia vaccine in aged animals. The results demonstrated that aged mice could produce antibodies against antigens similar to normal mice, leading to a significantly high survival rate against pneumonia infection. These findings suggest that the function of aging immunity is not completely regressed and that the utilization of appropriate immune boosters can enhance the efficacy of vaccines for the elderly. This insight is particularly pertinent as free vaccines for influenza and pneumonia are administered to the elderly annually, yet they have been known not to significantly reduce the fatality rate from the actual infections. The persistent call for immune boosters capable of inducing immunosenescence demonstrates an ongoing need, particularly in light of new infectious diseases that are anticipated to emerge periodically. The emphasis on such additional research holds considerable importance for preparing and responding to future infectious threats. Therefore, TLR5 emerges as a beacon of hope in the field of immunology and gerontology. The escalating interest in its potential to boost immunosenescence reflects the promise it holds. As research progresses, we anticipate that TLR5-targeted interventions will significantly influence the infectious disease market and contribute to a future where the elderly population enjoys enhanced immunity and quality of life.

Summary

Exploring the immune system of centenarians is essential in uncovering aging mysteries and developing strategies for a healthier lifespan. Understanding mechanisms that enhance aging immunity is crucial, aiding in the development of immune boosters to fortify defenses as we age, addressing the societal imperative due to the growing aging population and increased age-related diseases. Research in this field is key to discovering factors related to aging, health, and longevity, allowing for effective management of age-related issues, and revealing the secrets to centenarians' longevity and health. Further research and innovative developments are essential for individuals seeking healthy aging. The pursuit of this knowledge aims not only to extend life but to enrich it, ensuring vitality and wellness in our later years. Integrating insights from centenarian immunity and exploring new immune boosters are steps towards a future where aging signifies strength and resilience, not vulnerability.

References

- Biagi E, Franceschi C, Rampelli S, Severgnini M, Ostan R, *et al.* Gut microbiota and extreme longevity. Current Biology 2016;26(11):1480-1485.
- Bulati M, Buffa S, Candore G, Caruso C, Dunn-Walters DK, *et al.* B cells and immunosenescence: a focus on IgG+ IgD− CD27−(DN) B cells in aged humans. Ageing research reviews 2011;10(2):274-284.
- Chambers ES, Akbar AN. Can blocking inflammation enhance immunity during aging?. Journal of Allergy and Clinical Immunology 2020;145(5): 1323-1331.
- Chung HY, Cesari M, Anton S, Marzetti E, Giovannini S, *et al.* Molecular inflammation: underpinnings of aging and age-related diseases. Ageing research reviews 2009;8(1):18-30.
- Colonna-Romano G, Buffa S, Bulati M, Candore G, Lio D, *et al.* B cells compartment in centenarian offspring and old people. Current Pharmaceutical Design 2010;16(6):604-608.
- Gurinovich A, Song Z, Zhang W, Federico A, Monti S, *et al.* Effect of longevity genetic variants on the molecular aging rate. GeroScience 2021; 43(3):1237-1251.
- Karagiannis TT, Dowrey TW, Villacorta-Martin C, Montano M, Reed E, *et al.* Multi-modal profiling of peripheral blood cells across the human lifespan reveals distinct immune cell signatures of aging and longevity. EBioMedicine part of The Lancet Discovery Science 2023;90:104514.
- Komaki S, Nagata M, Arai E, Otomo R, Ono K, *et al.* Epigenetic profile of Japanese supercentenarians: a cross-sectional study. The Lancet Healthy Longevity 2023;4(2):e83-e90.
- Lens-Pechakova LS. Centenarian rates and life expectancy related to the death rates of multiple sclerosis, asthma, and rheumatoid arthritis and the incidence of type 1 diabetes in children. Rejuvenation Research 2016; 19(1):53-58.

- Lim JS, Nguyen KCT, Nguyen CT, Jang IS, Han JM, *et al.* Flagellin-dependent TLR 5/caveolin-1 as a promising immune activator in immuno-senescence. Aging Cell 2015;14(5):907-915.
- Moskalev A, Stambler I, Caruso C. Innate and adaptive immunity in aging and longevity: the foundation of resilience. Aging and disease 2020;11(6): 1363-1373.
- Ogata K, An E, Shioi Y, Nakamura K, Luo S, *et al.* Association between natural killer cell activity and infection in immunologically normal elderly people. Clinical and Experimental Immunology 2001;124(3):392-397.
- Rubino G, Bulati M, Aiello A, Aprile S, Gambino CM, *et al.* Sicilian centenarian offspring are more resistant to immune ageing. Aging clinical and experimental research 2019;31:125-133.

- Rubino G, Bulati M, Aiello A, Aprile S, Gambino CM, *et al.* Sicilian centenarian offspring are more resistant to immune ageing. Aging clinical and experimental research 2019;31:125-133.

- Sato Y, Atarashi K, Plichta DR, Arai Y, Sasajima S, *et al.* Novel bile acid biosynthetic pathways are enriched in the microbiome of centenarians. Nature 2021;599(7885):458-464.
- Zhavoronkov A. Geroprotective and senoremediative strategies to reduce the comorbidity, infection rates, severity, and lethality in gerophilic and gerolavic infections. Aging (Albany NY) 2020;12(8):6492-6510.
- Zhou L, Ge M, Zhang Y, Wu X, Leng M, *et al.* Centenarians alleviate inflammaging by changing the ratio and secretory phenotypes of T helper 17 and regulatory T cells. Frontiers in Pharmacology 2022;13:877709.

Chapter 13

Genetics of Korean Centenarians

Sung Sun Kim

Introduction

The genetics of aging and longevity is a complex and exciting field of research that seeks to understand the genetic factors that influence how an individual lives and ages. Here are some key points about genetics as they relate to aging and longevity.

Genetics plays an important role in determining an individual's potential lifespan. The genetic code contained in DNA contains information that affects various aspects of aging, including susceptibility to age-related diseases and the speed of aging. Some genes have been found to have a direct impact on lifespan. One of the best-known longevity-related genes is the *APOE* gene, which appears in several variants (alleles). The *APOE4* allele is associated with an increased risk of Alzheimer's disease and may affect lifespan. Other genes such as *FOXO3A*, *SIRT1*, and *MTOR* have also been linked to longevity [Choi YH *et al.*, 2003, Reinvang I *et al.*, 2013].

Telomeres are repetitive DNA sequences at the ends of chromosomes that protect them from breakdown. These tend to shorten each time a cell divides and are associated with aging [Rudolph KL *et al.*, 1999]. The telomerase enzyme can maintain or even lengthen telomeres, potentially extending cell lifespan. Genetic variations in telomerase and telomere maintenance genes can affect aging and lifespan.

Genetic mutations and DNA damage accumulate over time and contribute to aging. Genes involved in DNA repair and maintenance, such as *BRCA1*, *BRCA2*, and *WRN*, are important for preserving genetic integrity. Epigenetic modifications, such as DNA methylation and histone modification, can influence gene expression and age-related changes. Epigenetic clocks, which measure these modifications, have been developed to estimate biological age.

Caloric restriction (reducing calorie intake without malnutrition) has been shown to extend lifespan in various organisms [Rebrin I *et al.*, 2011]. Genetic pathways like mTOR and AMPK are involved in the response to caloric restriction and can influence longevity. Chronic inflammation is associated with many age-related diseases. Genes related to the immune system, such as *IL-6*, *TNF*-alpha, and *NLRP3*, can play a role in aging [de Gonzalo-Calvo D *et al.*, 2010].

Studies of twins and families have shown that genetics can significantly impact longevity. Identical twins, who share nearly identical genetic makeup, often have similar lifespans compared to fraternal twins. It's important to note that genetics is just one piece of the puzzle. Lifestyle factors, environmental influences, and chance events also play crucial roles in aging and longevity. The interplay between genetics and these external factors is complex and not fully understood. Genetic testing services like 23andMe and AncestryDNA can provide insights into certain genetic factors related to aging and health.

However, these results should be interpreted in consultation with a healthcare professional.

Why Genetic Research on Very Old People is Important

Genome research on the very elderly population is crucial due to its potential to provide insights into the genetic factors underlying the longevity and age-related diseases prevalent in this unique demographic group. The study of the genomes of very elderly individuals is essential to identify specific genetic variations associated with exceptional longevity. By comparing the genetic profiles of long-lived individuals with those who have average lifespans, researchers can pinpoint genetic factors that may contribute to a longer and healthier life. Aging is often accompanied by an increased risk of a variety of age-related diseases, including Alzheimer's disease, cancer, and cardiovascular disease. Genomic studies can reveal genetic signatures and mutations associated with these diseases, aiding in early diagnosis, risk assessment, and development of targeted treatments.

Understanding the genetic basis of longevity and age-related diseases may facilitate the development of precision medicine approaches [Au R *et al.*, 2019]. People can use this information to create more effective healthcare strategies by customizing medical treatments and interventions based on a person's unique genetic profile. Genomic studies can reveal genetic biomarkers associated with aging and age-related diseases and can inform the development of pharmaceuticals targeting age-related diseases. These biomarkers can serve as diagnostic tools, identifying individuals at higher risk for certain conditions and enabling early intervention. Medical professionals can utilize genetic data to assess an individual's genetic predisposition to age-related diseases. This personalized risk assessment can guide patients and healthcare providers to make informed decisions regarding preventive measures and screening protocols.

Genomic studies of the very elderly may help us better understand population health trends. This may help identify genetic factors that may be unique to the Korean population and inform public health policies to improve the overall health and well-being of older adults.

Genomic studies of Korea's very elderly population are important because they offer the potential to reveal genetic markers, pathways, and therapeutic targets associated with longevity and age-related diseases. This knowledge could lead to advances in personalized medicine, diagnostics, and treatments that improve the health and quality of life of older adults in Korea and abroad.

History of Genome Research in the Supercentenarians

Research into longevity began in the 1930s when researchers observed that calorie restriction in mice and rats increased their lifespan. In the 1950s and 1960s, Medawar's mutation accumulation theory, Williams' antagonistic pleiotropy hypothesis, and the Hayflick Limit were proposed [Campisi J *et al.*, 2019]. Since the late 1980s, studies using *C.elegans* have reported that specific genes are related to lifespan. Even after 2000, research on calorie restriction continued, with studies showing that *TOR* is involved and studies showing that calorie restriction in rhesus monkeys is associated with extended lifespan. In 2009 and 2013, there were studies showing that rapamycin and metformin extend mouse lifespan, and in 2016, the TAME (Targeting Aging with Metformin) trial began in humans(Table 13-1).

Table 13-1. History of genome research of aging

Period	Research
1930s	Calorie restriction studies
1950~60s	Medawar's mutation accumulation theory, Hayflick limit proposal
1980~90s	Gene study using *C.elegans* and yeast
2000~	Expansion of genetic study to mammalians and humans
2010~	TAME trial in humans and senolytics clinical trial

Genomic research related to longevity can be broadly divided into studies using gene level, tissue level, and single-cell sequencing. Genes found to be significant in the Genome-Wide Association study include *APOE*, *APOC1*, *TOMM40*, *CAMKIV*, *OTOL*, *MINPPI*, and *FOXO*3a, and these studies used sets consisting of discovery samples (discovery phase) and replication samples (validation phase) [Murabito JM *et al.*, 2012]. A study comparing transcriptomes of donor tissues to compare "healthy" and "common" aging was recently reported and showed that gene sets related to cholesterol and homocysteine levels were significantly downregulated in "healthy" aging [Zeng L *et al.*, 2020]. Recently, a study was reported that revealed through single cell sequencing that the immune system of supercentenarians is different from that of the elderly. The authors reported that cytotoxic CD4 T cells were increased through single-cell transcriptome profiling of peripheral blood mononuclear cells from supercentenarians and control groups [Hashimoto K *et al.*, 2019].

Aging-related Genomic Research Conducted in Korea

In the case of Koreans, unlike Western studies, Choi YH *et al.*, reported that neither the *ACE* nor *APOE* genes were significantly related to longevity [Choi YH *et al.*, 2003]. However, the *APOE* e4 allele is still associated with dementia, even in people over 100 years of age. [Kim, KI *et al.*] conducted a study on the effect of p22phox C24T polymorphism, an important component of NAD(p)H oxidase, an important oxidative stress source, on cardiovascular aging. Although no significant difference was identified in the p22phox genotype frequency according to the subject's age, a significant association was reported between the p22phox genotype and hypertension [Kim KI *et al.*, 2007., Kim DJ *et al.*] compared centenarians and controls to determine the relationship between *MLH1*, one of the DNA mismatch repair genes, and longevity. They observed that certain *MLH1* haplotypes were found significantly more in centenarians [Kim DJ *et al.*, 2006]. Recently, a study on the gut microbiota of longevity people was published, and the authors compared the gut microbiota of centenarians, older people, and adults in a longevity village with those of urban older people and adults. In centenarian villages, *Firmicutes* was relatively abundant and *Bacteroidestes* was found to be relatively low [Kim BS *et al.*, 2019]. Although additional research is needed on the function of each microbial group, it has been confirmed that centenarians' intestinal flora is different, making it possible to assume that their immune status and intestinal environment will be different.

Summary

As mentioned earlier, genomic research on longevity is expected to be helpful in personalized approaches and management of diseases caused by aging, the development of related drugs, and the development of diagnostic, therapeutic, and prognostic markers for degenerative diseases. In both genetics and microbiome research for longevity or healthy aging, collaboration with experts in genetics, microbiology, bioinformatics, and statistics is essential to ensure research success. Additionally, securing funding, maintaining well-documented research protocols, and staying up to date on the latest technologies and methodologies are critical to successful research into longevity and healthy aging.

References

- Au R, Ritchie M, Hardy S, Ang TFA, Lin H. Aging Well: Using Precision to Drive Down Costs and Increase Health Quality. Adv Geriatr Med Res. 2019;1:e190003.
- Campisi J, Kapahi P, Lithgow GJ, Melov S, Newman JC, Verdin E. From discoveries in ageing research to therapeutics for healthy ageing. Nature. 2019;571(7764):183-192.
- Choi YH, Kim JH, Kim DK, Kim JW, Kim DK, Lee MS, Kim CH, Park SC. Distributions of ACE and APOE polymorphisms and their relations with dementia status in Korean centenarians. Journals of Gerontology Series a-Biological Sciences and Medical Sciences. 2003;58(3):227-231.
- de Gonzalo-Calvo D, Neitzert K, Fernandez M, Vega-Naredo I, Caballero B, Garcia-Macia M. Suarez FM, Rodriguez-Colunga MJ, Solano JJ, Coto-Montes A. Differential inflammatory responses in aging and disease: TNF-alpha and IL-6 as possible biomarkers. Free Radic Biol Med. 2010;49(5):733-737.
- Hashimoto K, Kouno T, Ikawa T, Hayatsu N, Miyajima Y, Yabukami H, Terooatea T, Sasaki T, Suzuki T, Valentine M, Pascarella G, Okazaki Y, Suzuki H, Shin JW, Minoda A, Taniuchi I, Okano H, Arai Y, Hirose N, Carninci P. Single-cell transcriptomics reveals expansion of cytotoxic CD4 T cells in supercentenarians. Proc Natl Acad Sci U S A. 2019;116(48): 24242-24251.
- Kim BS, Choi CW, Shin H, Jin SP, Bae JS, Han M, Seo EY, Chun J, Chung JH. Comparison of the Gut Microbiota of Centenaria ns in Longevity Villages of South Korea with Those of Other Age Groups. Journal of Microbiology and Biotechnology. 2019;29(3):429-440.
- Kim DJ, Yi SM, Lee SY, Kang HS, Choi YH, Song YW, Park SC. Association between the MLH1 gene and longevity. Hum Genet. 2006; 119(3):353-354.

- Kim KI, Na JE, Kang SY, Cho YS, Choi DJ, Kim CH, Kim HS, Oh BH, Choi YH, Kwon IS, Park CS. Impact of NAD(P)H oxidase p22 (phox) gene polymorphism on vascular aging in Korean centenarian and nonagenarian. International Journal of Cardiology. 2007;123(1):18-22.
- Murabito JM, Yuan R, Lunetta KL. The search for longevity and healthy aging genes: insights from epidemiological studies and samples of long-lived individuals. J Gerontol A Biol Sci Med Sci. 2012;67(5):470-479.
- Rebrin I, Forster MJ, Sohal RS. Association between life-span extension by caloric restriction and thiol redox state in two different strains of mice. Free Radic Biol Med. 2011;51(1):225-233.
- Reinvang I, Espeseth T, Westlye LT. APOE-related biomarker profiles in non-pathological aging and early phases of Alzheimer's disease. Neurosci Biobehav Rev. 2013;37(8):1322-1335.
- Rudolph KL, Chang S, Lee HW, Blasco M, Gottlieb GJ, Greider C, DePinho RA. Longevity, stress response, and cancer in aging telomerse-deficient mice. Cell. 1999;96(5):701-712.
- Zeng L, Yang J, Peng S, Zhu J, Zhang B, Suh Y, Tu Z. Transcriptome analysis reveals the difference between “healthy” and “common” aging and their connection with age-related diseases. Aging Cell. 2020;19(3):e13121.

PART IV

CASE STUDIES OF KOREAN CENTENARIANS

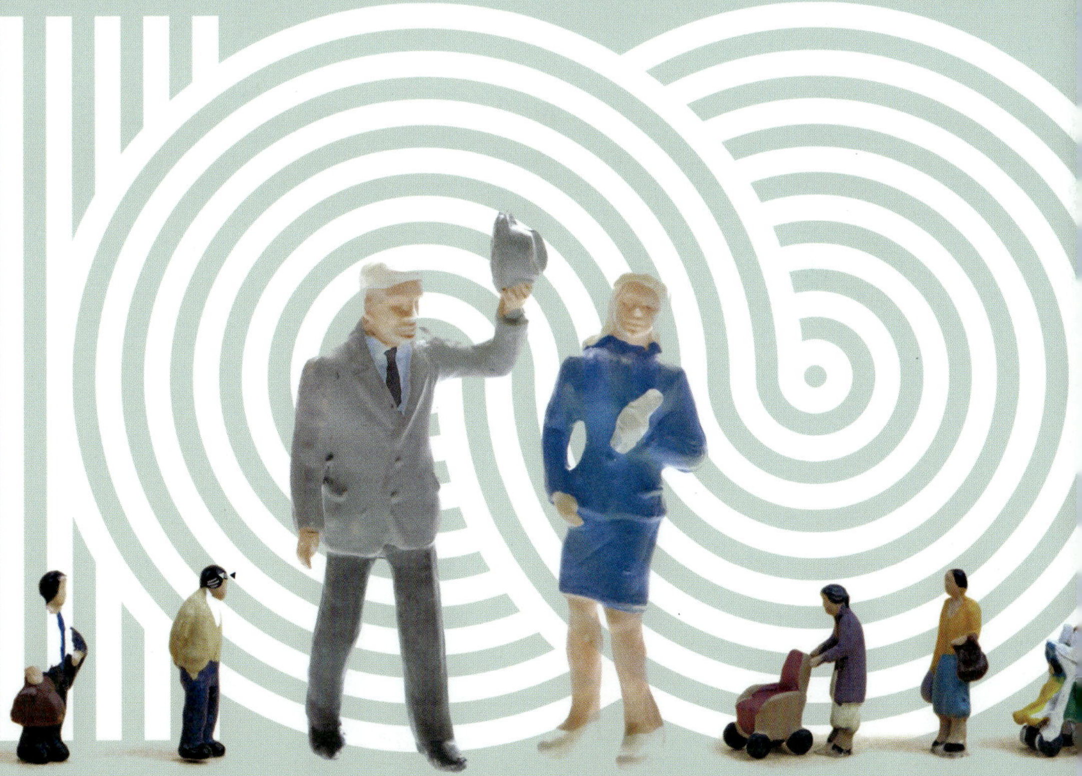

Chapter 14

Special Cases of Centenarians in the GuGokSunDam Longevity Belt

Sang Chul Park, Kwangsung Park, and Jeonghwa Lee

A Sketch of Centenarians in the GuGokSunDam Region 20 Years Ago

A centenarian whom a Time magazine reporter admires

When a reporter from Time magazine approached us for a special feature on Asian longevity, we provided him with an array of materials. These included biographies of centenarians and introductions to counties like Sunchang, Damyang, Gokseong, and Gurye, known for their higher ratio of centenarians. Yet, the representative centenarian from Korea highlighted in Time's July 21, 2003 issue was Mrs. Park BD, age of 100, from Banghwa Village, Gurim-myeon, Sunchang Gun County(Figure 14-1).

Mrs. Park, as chosen by the Time magazine reporter, was an exceptional individual. When our research team planned to visit, the village chief advised we needed to bring a bottle of alcohol, hinting at her fondness for the drink. When visiting centenarians, we usually prepare a gift bundle of vitamins and cookies, never thinking of alcohol as a present. Heeding the advice, we purchased two bottles of the Korean drink Soju.

Upon arrival, we met a fair-skinned older woman. Engaging her in conversation proved challenging, especially when she revealed the recent loss of her 79-year-old son, which left her disheartened and wary of strangers. To ease the tension, we offered her a glass of alcohol. To our surprise, she downed it effortlessly and encouraged us to partake. Even the village chief and the neighbors were prompted to drink at her insistence. Her active action on alcohol embarrassed us. Therefore, we were a little bit puzzled as to whether she could be the real centenarian. But by cross-referencing her age with her children and neighbors, we could confirm her age.

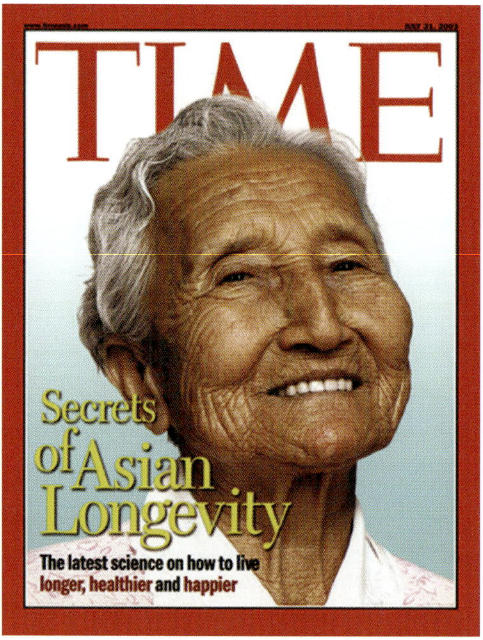

Figure 14-1. Korean longevity was for the first time globally introduced in Time's July 21, 2003 issue.

The topic of her late son brought her to tears. She lamented that he had passed before her at the age of 80. During our survey, a light rain fell, and her mood suddenly shifted. She energetically directed her 75-year-old daughter-in-law to dry the herbs. Watching her do the jobs, Mrs. Park praised her daughter-in-law profusely, stating she couldn't imagine life without her.

Mrs. Park's daily alcohol indulgence indeed intrigued the Time reporter. At the end of his visit, he asked us: “Do you think Korean traditional drinks, soju or Mageoli contribute to longevity?” After all, Mrs. Park, who maintained impressive health, lived up to the age of 107.

A centenarian living with dignity and consideration for family

In many cultures, it's customary to relinquish larger spaces to the younger generation as one ages, often resigning oneself to smaller rooms or areas near. In our travels across Korea, documenting the lives of centenarians, a common thread emerged – almost none lived with their families yet retained the house's main room. However, an exception came to light during a visit to Gokseong-gun.

Entering the house of a 102-year-old lady, Mrs. Ha HS, we were taken aback. The matriarch was comfortably settled in the home's largest room, while her second son, aged seventy-five, and his wife occupied a smaller space. When asked about the unusual arrangement, the son stated, “My mother deserves the big room.” There was no need for further justification.

We learned more about this exceptional lady as we interacted with the family. Still strong and healthy, she could thread a needle without assistance, her eyes sparkled with clarity, and she maintained a diverse diet without fuss. She was optimistic and rarely lost her temper. However, there was a singular quirk that amused her family. The lady had a strong penchant for alcohol. When her grandchildren gifted her money, she'd occasionally spend it on the drink, hiding it in her room. It became a light-hearted game between her and her son, who would find and dispose of the bottle, only to discover she had hidden away in fear of health problems.

Towards the end of our survey, the lady made a heartfelt request. She asked us to convey her appreciation for her daughter-in-law as we left. It was evident that even in her advanced age, she continued to play a pivotal role in the family dynamics. Observing this centenarian leading her household with grace, dignity, and a playful spirit made us see the beauty and pride of age.

A centenarian who checks on her old children every day

It is rare to find centenarians to have all their children around them. Even more unimaginable is that a centenarian holds all their offspring to be present or live together in one village. Yet, we encountered one remarkable centenarian: Mrs. Cho AJ, in Muksa-dong-myeon, Gokseong-gun.

Now 104, her hearing is diminished, but she remains spirited. Her eyes are sharp enough to thread a needle. While her son described her as occasionally impatient and demanding, she generally exudes positivity and energy, always mindful not to overeat.

Mrs. Cho has three sons and two daughters. Two daughters are married and reside outside of the village, while three sons live within the village. The ages of her sons range from 76 to 68. During our stay, all three sons sat attentively in their mother's presence. She pointed to a house about fifty meters away and said, “That's my second son's house.” She mentioned that she visits his house daily, checking the kitchen, lighting, and even resting in the main bedroom. However, she lamented being unable to check her youngest son's house since it's far in the village, separated by a stream. Despite this, all her sons, devoted to their mother, make it a rule to greet her daily whenever they are in the village.

When asked about the frequent visits from her sons, she softly replied, “I only get to see them every day. I miss them, even if it's just a day apart.” Her words conveyed profound emotion, emphasizing how a mother, even at a centenarian age, deeply misses her children in their seventies. As we prepared to leave, she added, “I hope my sons are blessed. They are irreplaceable to me.” The depth of her love and her sons' reciprocal respect transcends age, a testament to the enduring family bonds.

A centenarian who is favored by the town people

Many centenarians are outgoing and friendly by nature. Thus, neighbors frequently visit and care for them even when they live alone, especially in the countryside. This communal support often makes the emotional and daily lives of older people in the country much more vibrant and bearable compared to the isolated lives of those in the urban area.

On our visit to Buntong-ri Village in Yongmyeon, Damyang Gun, we were very much impressed by the unique layout of the town. A creek meanders through the village's heart, with all house gates facing it. This design makes it easy to spot residents strolling by and viewing those living in neighboring houses.

However, Mrs. Shin GS, at the age of 100, truly attracted our special interests. When we arrived at her house, we were met with an unexpected sight: a gathering of neighbors around her humble, albeit dilapidated, abode. Inside, half a dozen locals sat on the floor while others filled her yard, animatedly discussing various topics. Initially, we assumed our presence as a research group triggered it. Soon, we learned this was a regular occurrence. It was not because of our visit but because of her inconvenience. When questioned, they recounted how they began visiting her for comfort after Mrs. Shin injured her leg earlier in the year. This tradition persisted, transforming her home into the village's communal space despite the modern, well-constructed community center nearby.

As we delved into her history, it became apparent that life hadn't always been kind to Mrs. Shin. Gambling and alcohol had claimed the resources of her husband and children, leaving her primarily alone, except for occasional visits from her out-of-town daughter. Yet, her resilience and character were apparent. When a village issue arose, she took part voluntarily to intervene, solving matters personally. And if she ever received a gift or favor, she would reciprocate promptly. In case, vitamins were supplied from the health center, she paid back by weeding its lawns at dawn. She never let a good deed go unanswered.

Her selfless nature and unwavering spirit in adversity endeared her to the community. Having overcome numerous challenges with an indomitable will to thrive and an ever-present readiness to give back, Mrs. Shin might well represent an ideal symbol of successful longevity.

An example of a traditional long-live family: Up-4 and Down-4 generation family

Traditionally, in our society, there is a word depicting a long-lived family as members of the family should live out spans of up-four and down-four generations in continuance. This requires a person of longevity family to witness a life with their father, grand-father, great-grandfather, and subsequently with their son, grandson, and great-grandson. Yet, encountering such individuals of the long-lived family is very rare.

While visiting Uiam-ri in Gokseong-gun, we stumbled upon the village of Bonghyeon, marked by a menhir boulder bearing its name. With the main entrance under construction, our bus could not pass. However, the village chief we had contacted earlier arrived in a small car with the lady of our concern. She was a 100-year-old Mrs. Gong MR. Alert and lively, she effortlessly indulged in dialogue and humor. Her spirited song of "Myeongsasimni" was delightful. Yet, what truly astounded us was to discover that her parents lived to be 86 and 87 years old, and all her siblings, aged 94, 91, and 85, still resided in the same village. Mrs.Gong, the eldest, still attends to her younger siblings daily, expressing concern for their well-being. Observing their interactions exuded an ageless bond of sibling love. Their lineage, extending back to their great-grandfathers and forward to their great-grandchildren, felt like witnessing a quintessential Korean family. Their story encapsulated the essence of traditional longevity in our society.

A Sketch of the 2022 Centenarians in the GuGokSunDam Region

The master of self-care: a glimpse into Mr. Kim's life

Mr. Kim BD, at 105 years old, exemplified the health and vitality of an ideal centenarian. We had the chance to meet this remarkable gentleman residing in Gurye-eup. Upon our arrival, his daughter-in-law ushered us into their pristine yard, revealing a meticulously cared-for garden and then leading us to Mr. Kim's room.

A slender figure with a sturdy posture greeted us. Mr. Kim, impeccably dressed, extended a warm welcome. Though his wife had been gone for 13 years, the elaborate order of his home bore no trace of her absence. As he wore the glasses to read and answer our interview questions, his demeanor radiated self-assuredness in his intellect and well-being.

Mr. Kim has shared his home with his second son, a civil servant, for 36 years, yet remains the undisputed head of the household. This dominance extends to managing his finances, right down to the meticulous act of serving and marking rice portions. His leadership qualities are recognized beyond just his household; until age 100, he chaired the Senior Citizens' Association of the village.

Contrary to typical health advice, his daughter-in-law shared that Mr. Kim's diet includes foods often deemed unhealthy, such as spicy dishes, salty treats, and even ramen. Despite this, he remains disciplined in other areas, sleeping at 8 PM. and ensuring a two-hour walk, aided by a cane, after meals. At the slightest sign of health anomalies, he's proactive, seeking medical care in Gwangju and diligently following medication and supplement regimens. Such autonomy extends to his travels as well, as he independently takes bus trips to visit his daughter in Gwangju.

Active social engagement is another cornerstone of his vibrant life. When he visits the senior center, about 20 elderly individuals often offer him their seats and spend their leisure time playing card game (Hwatu) together. Here, he engages in leisurely games of fetch, a testament to his enduring physical agility. This spirited involvement safeguards Mr. Kim from isolation and fortifies his bond with his community.

Deep-rooted in his Catholic faith, Mr. Kim conveyed a profound sentiment. He often feels that "Everything is always good" and seldom finds himself enveloped in sorrow. However, his recent contemplations revolve around his mortality. While he believes in a peaceful afterlife with God, the idea of death instills fear in him. Throughout his life, he has cherished autonomy and longevity, yet the inevitability of death and his emotions toward it transcend age.

Family ties and care beyond blood: devotion of the caregiver

In the tranquil rural neighborhood of Gurye-eup, Gurye-gun, neat rows of clean laundry billow gently in the wind, stretching across a spacious yard. This yard, filled with a thriving vegetable garden and dominated by pumpkin vines, tells a story of dedication and familial love.

Awaiting our arrival, Mrs. Cho KD (100) sat ready to greet us in her room. As we entered, we were warmly received by all members of the family, her three sons, her eldest grandson with a disability, and a crucial household member, their caregiver.

Mrs. Cho's life story is full of resilience and dedication. She married a man 15 years younger than her, with whom she had four sons. At 52, she was obliged to move to Jinju to support her third son, who was left alone after a divorce. When the same son later moved back to Gurye for work in an orchard, she accompanied him. The grandson living with her, born to her eldest son, was once cared for by her during his younger days. A tragic accident later paralyzed him, taking back into her nurturing embrace. As they aged, their bond grew stronger, each relying on and assisting the other.

While in her prime, Mrs.Cho had to manage all the household chores and responsibilities. However, as age set in and she needed assistance, a noticeable gap in familial support arose. Thereafter, a caregiver intervened in their lives. She began caring for the family ten years ago, dedicating two hours daily thanks to the long-term care insurance system's inception. Beyond her professional obligations, she also handled the laundry for Mrs. Cho, her son and her grandson. Their relationship blurred the lines between caregiver and family, interacting with each other with the same endearment and trust.

Mrs. Cho's son fondly reminisced about her accomplishments, noting her graduation from Ewha Haktang, one of the most modern schools in a century ago. Despite her limited mobility, she remained proactive about her health. Until 2017, she traveled to Hadong to prepare herbal medicines. Her diet consisted of rice paired with seaweed and herbs, consumed slowly over 30 minutes. Hygiene was maintained through a weekly bathing service. While she steered clear of medications, she supplemented her diet with nutritional aids from the local health center. Her routine was regular, with sleep coming at around 8-9 PM and lasting undisturbed till morning. A strong desire to work and be active was evident. Even in sweltering summer weather, she'd immerse herself in tasks at her place or a neighbor's, including weeding or harvesting bamboo shoots.

Mrs. Cho proudly remarked during our conversation, “I walk everywhere.” Her deformed feet stand as a testament to her active younger days. She showcased her wheelchair, which she fondly refers to as the “silver car.” Her ability to independently maneuver it, meet friends, and visit senior centers attests to her physical strength and underscores the boost in her morale and overall quality of life.

Life-long continuing fantastic love story: the devotion of a husband

Upon visiting a couple in Gokseong Gun, we were greeted by a scene of a gray-haired gentleman and a demurely smiling lady, their hands intertwined. Gentleman Mr. Cho JH (103), reminiscing about their marriage at the young age of 20, quipped, “While some relationships don't last half a century, we're still here, holding strong.” Although he seldom verbalized his love or gratitude, his actions spoke volumes — like doing the dishes for his wife whenever she couldn't. The lady (age, name) fondly recalled how he had always been proficient at this chore, even during their early days.

Mr. Cho followed a disciplined routine, sleeping at 8-9 PM., waking up at 6 AM. to tidy the yard, and maintaining his physical activity. After meals, he'd stroll in the yard or venture outside, making almost daily visits to the village hall. A diet primarily consisting of local vegetables sustained him. He mentioned he never anticipated such a long life and never opted for dentures. Our urologist inquired about his urinary behavior. Hesitantly with embarrassment, he eventually told us that he had woken up to urinate twice during the night.

He was admired by most of the town people, often commenting, "It's a blessing to have such longevity, good health, and loving children." However, his perspective on life is humbler, valuing a peaceful departure that spares his children any distress over an extended life.

Reflecting on life's prime moments, he shared his fondness for his younger days when he toiled and led a simple life without specific hobbies. His wife, with limited mobility, now requires assistance and is under the care of a level 3 nursing facility, aided by a caregiver. Their eldest son, a retired police officer, also plays an active role in their caregiving, especially over weekends. Historically, caregiving was seen as a woman-centric role, typically assumed by wives, daughters, or daughters-in-law. However, this narrative needs to be corrected, as evidenced by the increasing involvement of sons in caregiving tasks. Additionally, the functional and caring nature of the centenarian grandfather has allowed the couple to lead independent lives without leaning heavily on external care facilities or assistance.

Our meeting concluded with a heartfelt farewell as the centenarian couple awaited our departure, their presence and demeanor reminiscent of a poignant film scene.

Centenarian leadership: the boss of senior community facility

Recently, the notion of centenarians residing in senior living facilities has become increasingly common. Two decades ago, Korean seniors predominantly lived in their own homes, surrounded and supported by their families. However, with the introduction of long-term care insurance and the proliferation of senior care facilities, the elderly living landscape has greatly shifted.

We have met a spirited 104-year-old, Mrs. Lim YO, who resides in a specialized elderly care facility in Pungsan-myeon, Sunchang-gun. On our visit, as we strolled down the hallway and entered her communal living space, we noticed a living room ringed by individual rooms. Several seniors sat on sofas, engrossed in TV program. In her wheelchair beside the couch, lady Lim might have appeared small, but her presence was undeniable. At our entrance, she initially observed us in silence. Soon, she greeted us with a beaming smile, a thumb up, and declared proudly, “I'm the big boss here!” She enthusiastically recalled her days of vitality, when performed the famous song “Why do you call me” by Mr. Song Chang-sik in a national competition.

Mrs. Lim had one son and four daughters. She lived with her eldest son and his wife, maintaining her health till the age of 92. Thereafter, following a stroke and subsequent surgery, her health began to decline. Years later, because of her son's health deterioration due to kidney dialysis complications, she was obliged to transfer to the nursing home. Though her eldest son passed away a few years after, her remaining children shielded the truth from her, fearing the trauma might inflict her. Additionally, she remained unaware of her recent diagnosis of lung cancer, since family did not informed it to her.

Mrs. Lim is in the early stages of dementia, with occasional mood swings but mostly coherent cognition. She cherishes company, often addressing caregivers affectionately as "nurses", particularly about receiving greetings upon their entry. Her temper can be short, leading to occasional squabbles with fellow residents. It was said that the wheelchair the lady occupied was reserved for her. So, in the absence of other seniors, she would confidently claim that seat. Proud of her centenarian status, she often proclaims, "Being the oldest, I expect to be greeted first, fed first." After the interview, as we bid her farewell, the lady appreciated with somewhat exaggerated gestures and voice. 'Thank you for coming to visit an old grand-mother like me.'

Mrs. Lim exuded confidence, speaking with clarity and poise. Her two daughters, who live nearby, and her granddaughters play an instrumental role in her care, visiting frequently. Such familial care fortifies Mrs. Lim's sense of self-worth, evident in her vibrant expressions and words.

Rotating role of children for care of the centenarian

Most people who are 100 years old have several children. Traditionally, the eldest child, typically the son and his spouse, would take up the mantle of primary caregiver. However, we could observe a notable shift in that caregiving was not exclusive to the eldest but distributed among various siblings. One example is MR. Kim OH, a 101-year-old from Damyang.

Upon visiting Mr. Kim, his youngest daughter and son-in-law warmly greeted us. The tall, distinguished senior gentleman asked,

"What's the purpose of this research? Shouldn't you offer something in return? After all, it's my lunar birthday today." He went on to share his life journey: Marrying at 20 to his 18-year-old wife, they farmed and nurtured their two sons and three daughters together. They lived harmoniously for 77 years, showing their bond like sunflowers always turning towards each other. After his wife's demise four years ago, the children took it upon themselves to care for him.

Everyone of his children, except the second son, who was currently working, began visiting his father and stayed for a week in turn. Already four years have passed since the four children began taking weekly turns to stay at their father's house. This shared responsibility has not only eased the burden on any sibling but also bolstered the family's pride in their collective commitment. The healthy male centenarian appeared psychologically stable, maintaining a consistent life in his familiar home. He avoided nursing facilities and caregivers, sustaining social connections through regular visits with his children. This is truly one of the representative cases of the Aging-in-place strategy.

His daughter noted that his nutrition has improved and he remains mentally and physically robust, following a healthy diet, drinking in moderation, and maintaining an active lifestyle attributed to his years of farming. His impeccable vision allows him to read and write without glasses. When asked about his health, he confidently replied, "Today is good. Tomorrow is uncertain, so there's no point fretting over it."

Mr. Kim, once the head of the village, mentioned that he seldom visited the village hall after the age of 80. He believed it would not be proper to visit the village hall because the younger residents would feel compelled to stand up from their rest whenever he entered. Mr. Kim, an elder of the village, showed significant consideration for his fellow villagers. This is why people from the neighborhood frequently visit him, ensuring he doesn't feel lonely.

Official records confirmed he had lived independently for the past four years without support from the community. What enables this elderly gentleman, who's flagged for special attention, to continue his independent life? Even when interdependence has waned, familial support remains pivotal for older adults. Mutual respect and understanding can pave the way for harmonious relationships within the family, ensuring older adults are well looked after.

Chapter 15

A Special Case of the Medically Privileged Semisupercentenarian

Jeong Gwan Cho

It is well known that there are 3 types of centenarians: survivors, delayers, and escapers. The majority of centenarians are survivors or delayers who have developed dementia, heart problems, or cancer but have overcome the diseases. Here is a typical delayer case of semisupercentenarian woman who overcame a heart attack 3 times while she approached the age of 100 years.

Seo Gyun Kim was born in 1918 as an only daughter among her four brothers in Jusan-ri, Sapyeong-myeon, Hwasun-gun, Jeollanam-do, and received education in Korean language Hangul, Chinese characters, and calligraphy from her father who was the village private school (Seodang) teacher. At the age of 17, she got married to a man who was the only son of three generations and a year younger than her.

She and her husband worked tirelessly day and night, expanding their farmland and ensuring their children's education. However, at age of 46 in 1965, her husband passed away from a subarachnoid hemorrhage, leaving her to face everything alone. In around 1994, at the age of 75, she started to experience pain in her hip joint after walking or tending to her steep garden and had to take anti-inflammatory and pain medications once or twice a week(Table 15-1). As the pain worsened, she took the pill almost daily. Her son suggested surgery, but she refused, saying, "I don't have much time left. Why even consider surgery?" At the age of 78, she gave up gardening and instead went to a senior community center of the apartment complex at her fourth son's suggestion. Despite her firm refusal, the son asked her to visit just once, so she did. At first, she felt awkward, but soon she made friends and gained followers who called her 'big sister', so she commto the center daily.

In 2002, at the age of 83, she happened to measure her blood pressure with an automatic blood pressure monitor. She found it to be 170/100, so she started taking the antihypertensive pill(Table 15-1),

Table 15-1. Major medical history of Seo Gyun Kim

		Medical Problems	Management
75 (1994)		Hip osteoarthritis, both	NSAID
83 (2002)		Hypertension	Antihypertensive drug
88 (2007)		Hip osteoarthritis, both	Rollator walker with seat
91 (2010)	Sept.	Compression fracture, T10	Nerve block
	Nov.	T8, T9	Vertebroplasty
	Dec.	T7, T12	Conservative (back brace)
92 (2011, Jan.)		Cataract, both eyes	Surgery
95 (2014, Apr.)		Bow leg deformity	Wheel chair
96 (2015, May.)		Macular degeneration, Lt eye	Intraocular drug injection 5 times
97 (2016, Nov.)		Compression fracture, L1	Fosteo® SQ (2 years)
98 (2017, Nov.)		Myocardial infarction	Balloon for LAD, LCX arteries
99 (2018, Feb.)		Unstable angina	Stent for RCA artery
100 (2018, Nov.)		Myocardial infarction	Stent for LAD artery
103 (2022, Aug.)		COVID-19	Remdesivir

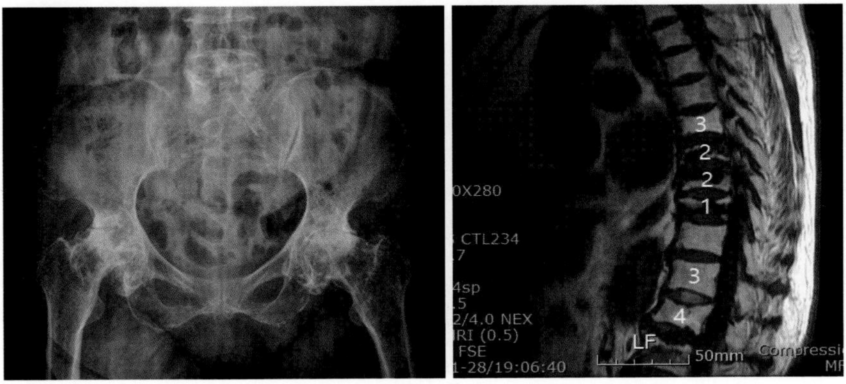

Figure 15-1. Orthopedic problems of the case. Left panel shows severe osteoarthritis in both hip joints. Right panel shows the sequence of compression fractures of the vertebra which is indicated by the number (1st: T10, 2nd: T8, 9, 3rd: T7, T12, 4th: L1).

but had no metabolic diseases such as diabetes and dyslipidemia. She visited the clinic for her hip joint pain again in 2005 at the age of 86 but was told that surgery was too risky due to her age, even though she had severe degenerative arthritis of the hip(Figure 15-1, Left panel). She continued non-steroidal anti-inflammatory drug (NSAID) medication and began using a cane. At the age of 88, walking to the center, which was about 300 meters away with a slight incline, was so painful that she had to take a break in the middle. So she used a Rollator walker with a seat that her son had bought for her. Her shoulders hurt as well, requiring intra-articular injection therapy several times. When she was young, she used to say, "Why save a body that will rot after death?" and used her body recklessly. As she got older, she realized that it was very stupid. She thought that she should save her body as much as possible for the coming Homo Hundred era.

In September, at the age of 91, she fell while turning her walker and suffered a compression fracture of her 10th thoracic vertebra(Figure 15-1, Right panel). She received nerve block treatment. In November of that year, she suffered compression fractures on the 8th and 9th thoracic vertebrae due to a shock from crossing a speed bump in a car. She underwent vertebroplasty and started taking osteoporosis medication. At this time, she realized how unbearable the pain of bones breaking could be. A month later, she suffered additional compression fractures in the 7th and 12th thoracic spine and was hospitalized, which left her relying on a wheelchair intermittently. She also developed cataracts and underwent surgeries at the age of 92 and 93.

In 2014, at the age of 95, she was baptized and given Clara as a baptismal name at a Catholic church. She was also rated as National Senior Long-term Care Insurance disability level 4, which authorized her to use long-term care services such as in-home bathing, home care, daycare, and a nursing home admission. At the age of 96, she had difficulty picking up side dishes with chopsticks and putting on shoes. She was diagnosed with macular degeneration. She received five rounds of intra-ocular injection therapy over the course of a year. Although her vision did not fully recover, the treatment helped her avoid complete blindness.

At the age of 97, she lost their eldest son on November 3rd, 2016. To make matters worse, she suffered from a compression fracture in the first lumbar vertebra (L1) on November 28th due to inadequate protective measures at her daycare center. She was hospitalized for 2 weeks at a university hospital and then transferred to a nursing hospital, where she stayed for a month. She refused the recommendation to extend hospitalization and decided to leave because she was asked to wear diapers despite no cognitive impairment. She often felt chest pain after returning to her last son's home from the hospital. She wondered if it was a kind of heartache because she was missing her darling eldest son, who had passed away just 2 months ago. Although her chest pain was not typical, she started anti-anginal medication just in case because angina pectoris should also be considered.

At the age of 98 (November 13th, 2017), after dinner, she experienced severe chest pain, so she put nitroglycerin under her tongue and her son drove her to the ER of a university hospital. She was diagnosed with acute myocardial infarction, and coronary angiography revealed that the right coronary artery (RCA) was completely blocked, and one of the two left coronary arteries was 90% blocked, while the other was 85% blocked. She received balloon angioplasty to widen it. After the treatment, symptoms improved slightly, but even a little exertion caused chest pain, and she felt that she would rather die than lead such a painful life. With her fourth son's insistence to undergo another procedure to open the completely occluded RCA, she decided to receive the procedure with the mindset that she had nothing to lose, even if she died. On February 27th, 2018(Figure 15-2). With all the efforts and techniques, they success

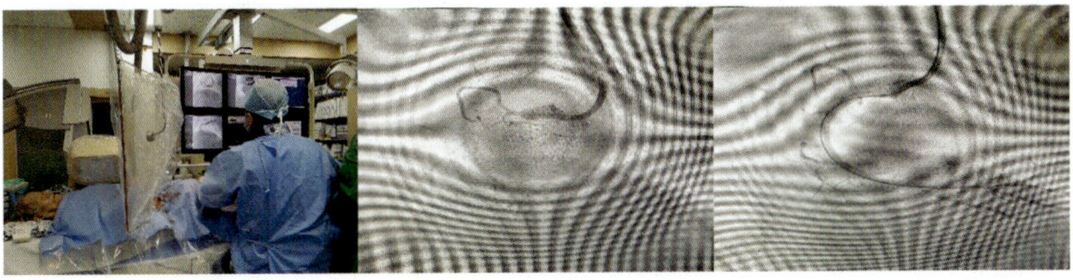

Figure 15-2. On February 27, 2018 (at the age of 99), second coronary artery intervention was performed to open up the chronic total occlusion of proximal right coronary artery (left and middle panel). The completely blocked artery was successfully recanalized using a special guide wire and then very good blood flow was restored (right panel)

fully opened the RCA and implanted a stent to hold it open. For the following several months, she lived comfortably as if the dark clouds had cleared. Still, symptoms of chest pain and shortness of breath occasionally returned even with full medication. Then, at midnight of November 21st, 2018, just before passing away, she was transported by 119 to the ER of CNUH(Figure 15-3, Left panel). She was diagnosed with acute myocardial infarction complicated with cardiogenic shock and received intensive care in the CCU to stabilize her medical condition. On November 22nd (one day before her 100th birthday), reopening and stenting for the completely occluded LAD coronary artery was successfully performed(Figure 15-3, Middle and Right panels). The next day, she ate a bowl of seaweed soup on her hospital bed to celebrate her 100th birthday. After the procedure, She felt no chest pain and breathed much easier, feeling like she was born again.

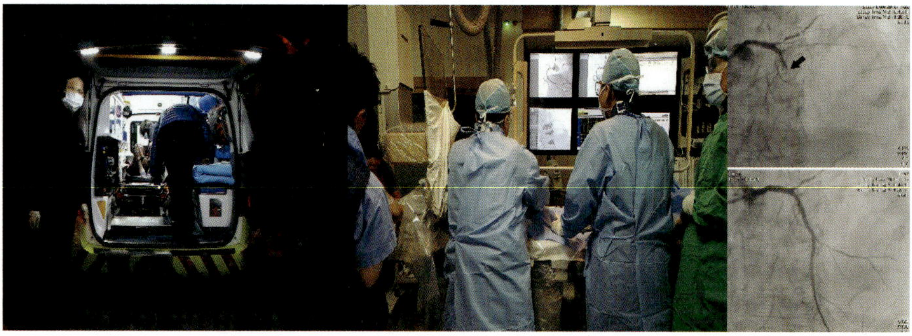

Figure 15-3. On November 21, 2018, she was taken to the ER of CNUH by a 119 ambulance because of severe ongoing chest pain and shortness of breath (left panel). Next day, she underwent third procedure (middle and right panel) to open complete blockage of the left anterior descending coronary artery (arrow in right upper panel) and implant a stent to prevent restenosis on the day before her 100th birthday.

PART IV

On August 17th, 2022, at age 103, she contracted COVID-19. Although the symptom was just like a common cold, she was admitted to the Univeristy Hospital for 3 days just in case. She recovered better than her fourth son in mid 60s, who transmitted COVID-19 to her.

As of 2023, at age 105, she lives with her fourth son and daughter-in-law. Although she has to use a walker to move around in the house, she can take care of herself regarding bowel movements and washing up. During the day, she goes to a senior daycare center, and in the evening, she watches TV with her son and enjoys the world news. On weekends, she happily spends time with her great-grandchildren, who come to visit. If she had not received the proper medical treatment, she would have become a resident of the afterlife long ago.

She emphasized, "My seven children were the reason for me to live as a young widow after losing my husband, and later they became the supporting power for me to live so long that I have never dreamed of. Although I moved around several of my children's homes, I never felt lonely because I lived with my children, and I have survived as a semi-artificial man by receiving timely treatments during a couple of crises. I sincerely appreciate all the medical staff who have cared for me and my children. I urge all seniors to seek medical treatment on time. Please do not hesitate to seek proper medical treatment because of old age.

PART V

PERSPECTIVES FOR FUTURE LONGLIVE SOCIETY

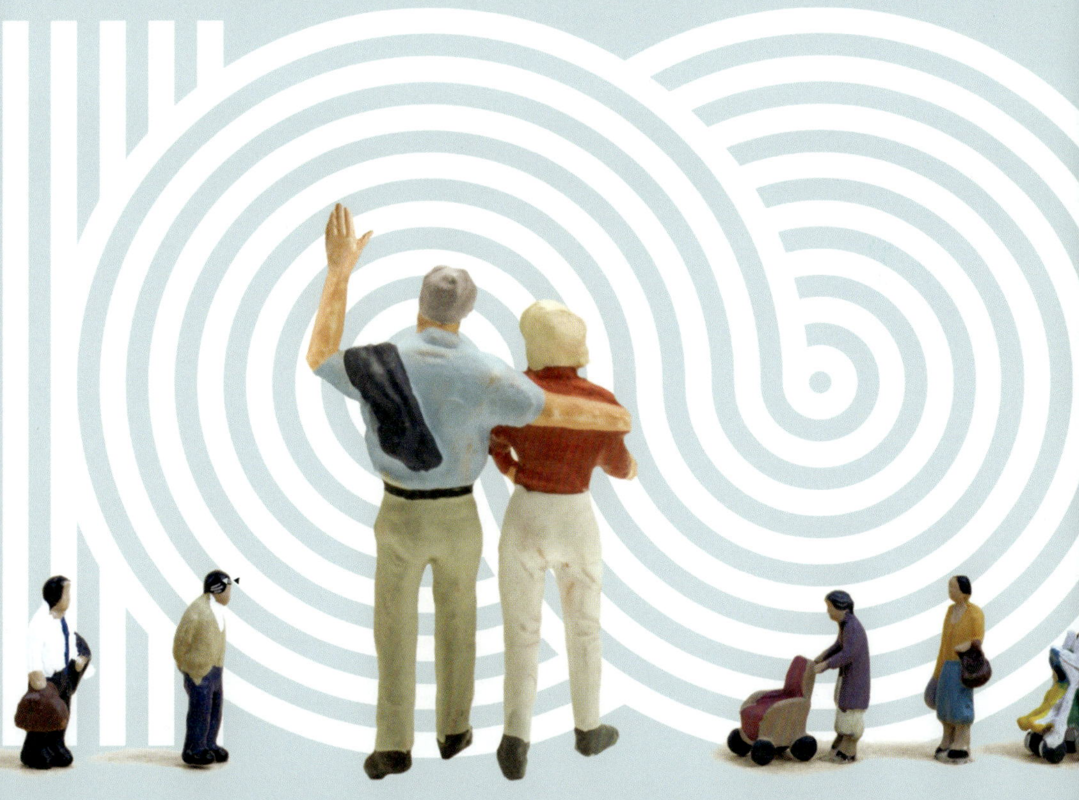

Chapter 16

Lessons from COVID-19 Crisis for New Normal in Future

Sang Chul Park

Longevity has always been a profound aspiration for humans. However, recently, debates have arisen questioning whether longevity is a bonus or an onus. Such debates stem from the inherent uncertainties associated with an aging society. Traditionally, longevity, wealth, nobility, health, and high honors are cited as the five blessings contributing to happiness, while short life, illness, worries, poverty, vice and weakness are the six extreme factors leading to unhappiness. The common and core element for both happiness and unhappiness relates to the length of lifespan. South Korea's recent ascension as the nation with the longest life expectancy was heartening but alarming the future. Further, a high mortality rate among older people in the COVID-19 pandemic brought special concerns. As we face this phenomenon of longevity, it's time to reestablish the paradigm of a super-aged society and consider solutions.

Changing World: New Dimension of Lifespan Extension

It was only after the 20th century that added an average of 30 years to human life expectancy. Advancements in the 20th century related to increasing lifespan include improved sanitation, electricity supply, and medical technology. In addition, enhancing living conditions, ensuring food safety, and liberating humans from diseases actualized the long-sought dream of an extended lifespan.

Interestingly, South Korea is expected to be the world's longest-living country in 2030 [Kontis *et. al.*, 2017]. Changes in life expectancy by country were projected for 35 developed countries, using 21 available forecasting models and analyzing statistics to predict future trends. In consequence, the average life expectancy of women in South Korea is anticipated to exceed 90 years for the first time in human history, and the average life expectancy of men will also exceed 84 years, making South Korea as the longest-lived country for both sexes. The economic improvements and the strengthening of social safety nets, including education have been listed as the responsible causes. Especially, the national improved nutrition through school lunches and nutrition education from elementary school onwards was emphasized to play the significant roles in extension of Korean longevity with the healthcare system, advanced medical technologies, and health insurance. Moreover, it was pointed out that obesity and hypertension rates are significantly lower than in other developed countries [Kontis *et. al.*, 2017]. This is the reason why South Korean longevity needs to be elaborated.

Temple model of human longevity

Human longevity cannot be explained in terms of just a few factors. According to Park's temple model of longevity, three components of the ground, pillars, and roof factors should be guarranted for human longevity as if building a temple [Park SC, 2012]. The ground factors are genes, gender, personality, socio-cultural and ecological conditions. The pillar factors are those of personal effort: exercise, nutrition, relationships, and engagement. Roof factors are welfare support systems, medical care, social security nets, and social infrastructures. This model implicates that longevity can be achieved not only by individual efforts but also by the public and environmental conditions. The private mechanism of longevity is dependent on individual genetic characteristics and life patterns, while the public mechanism of longevity is dependent on socio-cultural factors and local ecological characteristics. In order to live a long life, it is required to provide the sufficient conditions to do our best as individuals and the necessary conditions to fulfill our responsibilities as members of the community.

Scientific revolution in extension of individual longevity

For private mechanism of longevity, the life style factors such as nutrition, exercise, relationship and participation are listed. But these personal factors can be complemented and enforced with technical advancements. The traditional diets from longevity-rich regions like Okinawa and the Mediterranean as well as that of South Korea are gaining recognition as a longevity diet and the importance of eating habits of calorie restriction is highlighted [Park SC, 2016]. But for those who find it difficult to restrict food intake or enjoy eating, "calorie restriction mimetics" drugs that provide effects similar to fasting are being developed [Madeo *et al.,* 2019]. The regular exercise is strongly recommended for healthy longevity. But for those who cannot or do not like to exercise, or patients who need to be bedridden for extended periods due to injuries or illnesses, "exercise mimetics" providing the exercise effects without physical exercise are being developed [Pan *et al.,* 2017].

Further, there have been remarkable advancements in technology focused on strengthening individual physical abilities and enhancing the very phenomena of life [Park SC, 2021]. Assistive and augmentative technologies are used when muscles or sensory organs like eyes and ears become weak. Replacement technologies are focused on developing artificial organs and prosthetics to replace kidneys, hearts, livers, pancreas, and limbs. Especially, walking assistance devices and autonomous vehicles that can assist mobility are becoming essential items in an aging society. With advancements in robotics, communication means, and nanotechnology, these devices are becoming smaller, more functional, and enhancing biological functions while expanding the realms of physical activities both temporally and spatially.

Moreover, groundbreaking discoveries have transformed the landscape of biological aging itself. Technologies such as pluripotent stem cell induction and somatic cell nuclear transfer have introduced innovative avenues for reversing aging through artificial manipulation [Gurdon JB, 1962; Wilmut *et al.,* 1997: Takahashi & Yamanaka, 2006]. The application of parabiosis technology has spurred investigations into systemic factors capable of rejuvenating old organisms into a more youthful state [Conboy *et al.,* 2013]. Furthermore, selective methods for eliminating senescent cells have illuminated the technical potential for restoring youthful vitality [Kirkland & Tchkonia, 2020].

Despite controversies, the advancement of life science and technology has started to manipulate genes and transform the form and function of organisms. The method of improving in a more advantageous direction by repairing the genome in a recombinant manner by cloning the necessary genes has been already commercialized in crops and livestock as GMOs (Genetically Modified Organisms). Though, directly applying a genetic engineering system to humans raises serious ethical issues, it holds yet infinite potential [Park SC, 2019].

Another bold attempt is to cryogenically preserve patients who cannot be treated with current medical technology and then, when medical technology advances, to thaw and heal them. Cryopreservation is already used for various cells, bacteria, viruses, and other microbes, as well as the preservation of sperm and eggs. Successful births using frozen reproductive cells have been already widely accepted.

The scientific and technological advancements aiming at individual longevity have been dazzling in the 21st century. Dietary habits, exercise and wearable health devices have become common, while breakthroughs in life sciences, such as stem cell research, cloning, cryopreservation, xenografts, genetic engineering, and anti-aging remedies, pave the way towards a society of extreme longevity. These recent breakthroughs have challenged traditional notions of aging as irreversible and inevitable, opening up new possibilities for achieving ultimate control over the aging process and in consequence the extension of lifespan. However, while technological advancements may render mythic longevity achievable, they can drastically alter the framework of human relationships and might stray away from the traditional concept of happiness and quality of life.

Reconsideration required for public nature of longevity

It is necessary to redefine the longevity paradigm to achieve not just simple longevity, but a quality happy life in connection with public mechanism of longevity. There have been several important experiments on living conditions for the impact on human health and longevity by creating a perfect artificial environment. The notable Biosphere 2 project is one of them. A dome-shaped architectural structure that mimics the earth's ecosystems was prepared on the outskirts of Tucson, Arizona. Eight people, including doctors, scientists, and ordinary people, lived self-sufficiently for two years, researching and studying human life, lifespan, health, and changes in the earth's ecosystem. It was a large-scale environmental renovation project comparable to NASA's Apollo moon exploration project. Everything was meticulously planned for humans to live an ideal life harmoniously with nature, but it ended in significant failure. This experiment confirmed that environmental pollution and deranged human relationships would be the decisive obstacles in the future development of human society. Especially, the issue of human relationship is emerged as the most crucial and serious condition for future human society [Park SC, 2021].

The space in which humans live is not just a physical or chemical space but a social space where we must coexist harmoniously. However, with industrialization and informatization, human relationships have quantitatively expanded but have arguably regressed in terms of qualitative depth. To enhance human happiness and quality of life, it is essential to maintain an individual's health to its fullest and overcome novel epidemics and disasters through a robust societal system. We must ensure the safety of our living environment and overcome the adverse effects of environmental changes caused by both nature and humans. However, despite the advancement in science and technology, there are concerns about the quantitative and qualitative changes in human relationships, societal order, quality of life, and dignity.

Deterioration of relationships: Humanity has connected through direct physical contact as it grows and engages in social activities. Physical interactions enhance emotions and relationships, but indirect contacts due to the information revolution, though efficient and convenient, may reduce emotional exchange intensity, risking relationship persistence. A trade-off situation arises where concepts of convenience and efficiency prevail, sidelining human bonds of solidarity.

Generational conflict: While a generation typically spans around 25 years, this can change over time. Centenarians born in the late 19th century had a generational gap of only 20 years due to younger marriage ages, while currently, with later marriage ages, a generation spans over 30 years. Although genetics is passed down, the difference in birth era changes life patterns, culture, judgment criteria, and thinking due to political, economic, and social transformations experienced during growth. Hence, the zeitgeist changes for each generation, resulting in conflicts among generations.

Distortion of order: The rapid increase in the number of older people due to aging causes problems in the composition and operation of families and communities, requiring new ethics and order regarding generational responsibilities and roles. The advancement of science and technology maximizes individual abilities and enhances survival but can also lead to disparities based on region and class, potentially causing social inequality. Such inequality ultimately fosters resentment among residents, forms a divided society, and damages cohesion. Hence, establishing measures to address these changes in social structure and order is urgent.

Values and dignity maintenance: To live a life befitting of their nature, humans must lead a happy life that satisfies their values and dignity. When the UN compared the happiness indices of various countries, they reported where nations with higher happiness scores weren't necessarily wealthier but often poorer, which is designated as "Paradox of Happiness." In the future, what will be the solution to elevate human value and dignity, regardless of economic wealth or social systems? We must secure methods granting humans a sense of pride and value, providing societal worth.

Social support responsibility: Regardless of East or West, traditional societies were primarily based on a multi-generational family structure, where elderly care was a family matter, not a societal issue. With industrialization leading to urbanization, families have separated, transitioning to nuclear family societies, issuing elderly care in rural areas as a growing community issue. Subsequently, with the rise in divorce and single living, the shift towards one-person households has turned elderly care into a central topic requiring social intervention.

As societies age, they should become happier. However, the challenges of distorted human relationships, severe intergenerational conflicts, collapsing social orders, and shifting value systems are inevitable. Order and ethics are the foundation of long-lived communities, and if not adequately addressed, paradox of longevity, implicating the imbalance between lifespan extension and quality of life, can arise [Park SC, 2021]. The solution for these issues may come from the principles of the traditional community system in South Korea, consisted with promoting good deeds, correcting one's mistakes, maintaining social norms, and sympathizing during hardships.

Outbreak of COVID-19 Pandemic

The world's transition to a super-aged society has been marked by a dire warning. On January 7, 2020, the pathogen of an unexplained pneumonia outbreak in Wuhan, China, was identified as a new coronavirus. The WHO declared an international public health emergency on Jan 30, naming the virus as SARS-CoV-2 and unifying the nomenclature of the epidemic as COVID-19. On March 11, the WHO declared a pandemic to the global world. The lethality of the COVID-19 pandemic varies greatly by country, age, and gender. The differences between countries are due to differences in sanitation, health systems, lifestyles, and culture, and there are also large differences between men and women, with men's mortality rates higher than women's. But the difference in mortality rates by age is even stark. As of March 12, 2021, the Korean Centers for Disease Control and Prevention reported that only 7.5% of COVID-19 cases are in the 70s and 4.8% in the 80s, but 27.7% of deaths are in the 70s and 56.3% in the 80s, and the fatality rate is 6.5% in the 70s and 20.7% in the 80s, indicating an age-specific vulnerability that is 100-200 times higher than that of younger people under 40. In fact, in China and Italy, the mortality rate among confirmed COVID-19 cases is overwhelmingly higher among the elderly. The fact that the mortality rate is 1.5% in the 50s, 3.6% in the 60s, 8% in the 70s, and 14.8% in the 80s in China, and that 80% of COVID-19 deaths in China are among the elderly over the age of 60 and 90% of COVID-19 deaths in Italy are among the elderly over the age of 70, strongly raises the alarm about the severity of the elderly's health vulnerability to this infectious diseases. This exemplifies the paradox of longevity, where extreme age is a problem. In this COVID-19 pandemic, the warnings have been mainly directed to the elderly but not to children [Park SC, 2022].

New Normal for the Future Super-aged Society

The COVID-19 outbreak has not only exposed the threat of emerging infectious diseases to the world, but also highlighted how different countries and cultures are differently responding to this pandemic. It's tragic to see how even the most developed countries have been left with no facilities to house patients, and mass burials have been necessary to deal with the uncontrollable influx of dead bodies.

What is it about viral pandemics like influenza, SARS, MERS, and most recently COVID-19 that has caused such high mortality rates in the elderly? The decline in immunity with aging makes the elderly much more susceptible to infectious diseases and increases mortality rates. It is notable that the importance of lifestyle habit improvements has been underscored with over 95% of the fatalities from the COVID-19 pandemic having underlying health conditions like hypertension, diabetes, obesity, chronic pulmonary diseases, and cancer. In contrast, when centenarians are concerned, their mortality rate was reported to be only less than 5 %. It was a mystery while octogenarians' mortality is more than 20%, centenarians' mortality is far less. The answer could be derived from the simple fact that the medical characteristics of centenarians clearly show that majority of them are free from diabetes, hypertension, obesity and cancer, which are classified as life style diseases. In other words, the centenarians' life styles are healthy to overcome COVID-19 crisis (Park SC 2022). Thereby, solutions for future longevity society are explicit that prevention of diseases through lifestyle changes, supplemented by technological advancements, irrespective of race, age, or gender is essential. Further, COVID-19 crisis freshly brought out the time old issues of living conditions. The huge differences in mortalities among different countries suggest the significance of living conditions. Thereby, together with personal life styles, community culture, density and isolation are brought up as issues to be adjusted for new normal [Park SC, 2022]. The lessons from COVID-19 for new normal can be summarized as follows.

Life style correction: The COVID-19 crisis revealed that underlying conditions with high mortality rates, regardless of age, can be improved by lifestyle habits, emphasizing the crucial need for self-care efforts like regular exercise and proper diet as people age. Furthermore, solutions for aging societies must now prioritize the effort of self-reliance, learning and mastering how to live in familiar environments without becoming dependent on institutions like nursing homes. The essence of sharing and coexisting harmoniously with neighbors, based on self-care and self-reliance, is becoming increasingly evident. The pandemic suggests a movement where older people live independently, solving their problems and caring for themselves, regardless of age.

Community revival: We must actively address the potential paradoxes posed by longevity. Addressing the challenges of an aging society requires collective efforts, not just individual ones. Even if scientific advancements elevate individual capabilities, we cannot establish a truly happy, longevity society without a sense of community, maintained relationships, order, and dignity. Although longevity has always been a profound human aspiration, it loses significance without accompanying health and happiness [Park, 2010].

Aging in place: The issues with elder care facilities established in anticipation of an aging society became glaringly evident during the pandemic. Current living environments, which often involve close quarters, poor ventilation, and close contact, need reform. Systems like "Aging in Place," which encourage older people to live in their familiar environments, are essential. When care is required, a "Care in Place" system should be introduced, where medical professionals visit older people at their homes rather than hospitalization. Additionally, group homes and care farms, where older people live collectively and actively, are necessary to be provided.

Summary

The goal of humankind has always been to live longer and better, and in this quest, numerous shortcuts and tricks have emerged. But the inherent human desire to break the confines of time and extend life remains consistent. This desire has driven various scientific and technological advancements that have sequentially evolved our world. While humans have reached the pinnacle of evolution through adaptation, we're no longer merely adapting, but actively redesigning our species through science and technology. Therefore, to ensure that every individual is filled with health and happiness, alongside strengthening individuality, there's a pressing need to construct communities that maximize public spirit through social solidarity and cooperation. Especially in economic terms, to ensure that the society evolves into a low-cost longevity society and not a high-cost one, continuous efforts are needed from community members to become independent and maintain interdependent mutual respect and care. Through the COVID-19 pandemic, new normal principles for the community have been enlightened such as life style correction, community revival and aging-in-place. It is the lesson from the COVID-19 crisis to prepare in time for both the private independence and public interdependence of the future longevity society.

References

- Conboy MJ, Conboy IM, Rando TA. Heterochronic parabiosis: historical perspective and methodological considerations for studies of aging and longevity. Aging Cell. 2013;12(3):525-530.
- Fan W, Evans RM, Fan W. Exercise Mimetics: Impact on Health and Performance. Cell Metab. 2017;7;25(2):242-247.
- Gurdon JB. Adult frogs derived from the nuclei of single somatic cells. Dev. Biol. 1962;4:256-273.
- Kirkland JL, Tchkonia T. Senolytic drugs: from discovery to translation. J Intern Med. 2020;288(5):518-536.
- Kontis V, Bennett JE, Mathers CD, Li G, Foreman K, Ezzati M. Future life expectancy in 35 industrialised countries: projections with a Bayesian model ensemble. Lancet. 2017;389:1323-1335.
- Madeo F, Carmona-Gutierrez D, Hofer SJ, Kroemer G, Madeo F. Caloric Restriction Mimetics against Age-Associated Disease: Targets, Mechanisms, and Therapeutic Potential. Cell Metab. 2019;5;29(3):592-610.
- Park SC. Aging Revolution: Solutions to the Shock of Aging, Haso Publishing, 2010.
- Park SC. Comprehensive approach for studying longevity in Korean centenarians. Asian J Gerontol Geriatric. 2012;7:33-38.
- Park SC. Ethnic food for longevity pursuit: assessment of Korean ethnic food. J Ethnic Food. 2016;3:167-170.
- Park SC. Magnum Opus 2.0. Udeumji, 2019.
- Park SC. Longevity is a joint work of individuals and communities. Korean Academy Bulletin No. 333, 2021.
- Park SC. COVID-19 changed the Future of Longevity. Sigongsa, 2022.
- Takahashi K., Yamanaka S. Induction of pluripotent stem cells from mouse embryonic and adult fibroblast cultures by defined factors. Cell. 126, 2006; 663-676.

- Wilmut I., Schnieke A. E., McWhir J., Kind A. J. & Campbell K. H. Viable offspring derived from fetal and adult mammalian cells. Nature 385, 1997;810-813.

Chapter 17

Is there a Country for Old Men?

Jung Jae Lee

The Coen Brothers' 2008 film, "No Country for Old Men," with its alarming and evocative title, invoked memories that were anything but ordinary for my generation, which was primarily focused on economic development but not adequately prepared for retirement planning. In 2001, Seoul National University initiated a comprehensive research project led by Professor Sang Chul Park from the medical school. Its aim was twofold: to explore the exceptional nature of those reaching the age of 100 and to identify specific regions known for longevity. This multifaceted research examined various aspects of their lives, including health, genetics, dietary habits, family dynamics, social psychology, and environmental ecology. It centered its attention on regions renowned for their high population of centenarians, including Gurye, Gokseong, Suncheon, and Damyang, which became emblematic of the "GuGokSunDam longevity belt."

The study shed light on the paramount role of health insurance systems and minimum living support policies as the key determinants of longevity, thus highlighting the importance of national-level engagement within the community. Additionally, it unveiled some recurring traits among centenarians: they tend to be optimistic, possess life skills, maintain a strong sense of self-esteem, and adhere to regular lifestyles and exercise routines. Furthermore, the study stressed that achieving healthy longevity hinges on individuals' autonomy to make decisions and participate in livelihood activities, a perspective closely aligning with advanced longevity research conducted in countries such as Japan and the United States.

This research came into the spotlight and captured the attention of my generation which was ill-prepared for impending retirement. It sparked anticipation of follow-up studies and active government policies. Businesses hastily launched longevity products, the media aired shallow lifestyle specials, and an increasing number of individuals turned to rural living for a more comfortable retirement. Despite these initial reactions, the research failed to sustain momentum, and it became increasingly difficult to detect any coordinated government efforts or policies geared toward addressing the challenges of an aging society.

Fortunately, towards the end of last year, Chonnam National University conducted a follow-up study on centenarians in the "GuGokSunDam (Gurye, Gokseong, Suncheon, Damyang)" region. This research focused on centenarians in the same area, examining how physical and societal changes were influencing their longevity. Astonishingly, even within traditional rural communities, our long-standing tradition of multi-generational family cohabitation was undergoing a transformation. Back in 2001, a significant 68% of families in these traditional rural settings adhered to a multi-generational living arrangement. However, just last year, this figure plummeted to 32%, leading to a notable increase in elderly individuals living in isolation or seeking residence in nursing facilities. Adding to the concern is the fact that a significant proportion of this younger generation is also elderly. Inevitably, in the years to come, the remaining elderly population in rural areas is poised to encounter comparable circumstances. It's also becoming increasingly apparent that even the outskirts of aging cities are on the brink of mirroring a similar fate.

Over the past two decades, the birth rate has declined, but the overall population has not decreased. Society has aged, and family dynamics have undergone a significant transformation. The elderly dependency ratio, which was over 70% for all families, has rapidly dropped to the 20% range. In exchange, the public burden has increased from tens of trillions of Korean won annually to hundreds of trillions of won, raising concerns about the nation's economic growth. Especially with a decreasing youth population and an increasing elderly population, we are facing the grim prospect of the disappearing future caregiving generation. Due to the rapid increase in life expectancy, South Korea had little time to prepare for old age, leading to research suggesting that the so-called 'working silver' population (elderly people who continue to work) could be three to four times that of OECD countries. As a result, there is a frustrating clash between young and old for the same job opportunities, undermining the wisdom of the elderly and diminishing their dignity as human beings. Consequently, a new problem called generational polarization has emerged as a pressing issue in politics and society.

Irish poet William Butler Yeats, in his "Sailing to Byzantium," sang of a world where the wisdom of the elderly is disregarded, and action reigns supreme, stating, "That is no country for old men." Inspired by this sentiment, Cormac McCarthy wrote the novel "No Country for Old Men," which was later adapted into a film by the Coen Brothers. The author believes that the Coen Brothers emphasize the idea that “the elderly are not respected because they know but do not act” through the character Sheriff Bell (played by Tommy Lee Jones) in the movie. It is reminiscent of Dostoevsky's assertion that not acting despite knowing what is right is the true sin, as seen in “the virtue of a single onion root.”

The concept of creating a thriving aging society must present a fresh and promising opportunity. Traditionally, we have regarded the elderly as a burden, focusing on their care and support rather than recognizing their potential contributions. In contrast, advanced nations have embraced a different perspective, valuing the elderly and harnessing their experience as a source of new economic vitality. Amidst the challenges posed by an aging society at an unprecedented rapid rate, we must explore realms where experience and innovation intersect, including advanced technology and domestic industries, urban and rural environments, and the fusion of production and humanities. We should foster new industries that actively involve the elderly, and foster an aging society where they can work with dignity.

The younger generation should not fret over their own old age. This is the path to build a ‘Country for old men.’

Summary

In 2001, under Professor Sang Chul Park, Seoul National University delved into the exceptional characteristics of centenarians and identified the "GuGokSunDam longevity belt. Health insurance systems, community engagement, and autonomy in decision-making were central to longevity. Moreover, traits like optimism, regimented lifestyles, and self-esteem was recurrent among centenarians. The study resonated with a generation unprepared for retirement, prompting business and media attention. Yet, government responses dwindled over time. A subsequent study from Chonnam National University highlighted societal shifts: multi-generational cohabitation fell from 68% to 32% within two decades. As the younger generation also ages, fears grow over the caregiving future, with increasing economic burdens and the 'working silver' phenomenon leading to job market frictions. Amidst the societal challenges, literature and film, like "No Country for Old Men," underscore a disregard for elderly wisdom. The chapter advocates for a paradigm shift: instead of seeing the elderly as burdens, harness their expertise for economic rejuvenation, integrating advanced tech, and fostering industries that dignify aging. The goal is a society where all ages thrive.

Epilogue

For a Better Future with a Longer Lifespan

Sang Chul Park, Jeonghwa Lee and Kwangsung Park

The prospect of a longer lifespan presents both opportunities and challenges for individuals, communities, and societies as a whole. Since advancements in healthcare, technology, and socioeconomic factors contribute to an increased life expectancy, it becomes imperative to envision a future that embraces longevity while addressing its associated implications.

A longer lifespan calls for a shift in healthcare strategies towards preventive measures. Investing in regular health check-ups, promoting healthy lifestyles, and encouraging the early detection and treatment of diseases can significantly improve overall well-being and increase the quality of life in older adults.

Creating age-friendly environments that enable older adults to age in place, including accessible housing, transportation, and community services, is crucial for their independence, social engagement, and well-being. In addition, designing neighborhoods and public spaces that promote physical activity, social interaction, and access to healthcare services can enhance the overall quality of life.

Addressing the mental health challenges of older adults is essential for a better future with a longer lifespan. Implementing mental health programs, reducing the stigma of aging, and fostering supportive communities can improve mental well-being and ensure that advanced years can be characterized by a positive and fulfilling life.

Promoting intergenerational interactions and understanding is fundamental for fostering social cohesion and shared experiences across different age groups. Providing opportunities for older adults to actively participate in community activities, mentor younger generations, and contribute their wisdom and experiences can foster a sense of purpose and belonging.

Building robust social support networks that include family, friends, and community organizations is vital for individuals as they age. Encouraging strong social connections, volunteerism, and caregiving networks can provide emotional support, reduce social isolation, and enhance the overall well-being of older adults.

With longer lifespans, individuals may choose or need to work beyond traditional retirement ages. Creating flexible work arrangements, lifelong learning opportunities, and age-friendly work environments can ensure that older adults have the opportunity to continue to contribute to society, maintain financial security, and find fulfillment through work.

Recognizing the economic potential of older adults, societies should promote productive aging by leveraging their skills, knowledge, and experience. Encouraging entrepreneurship, providing retraining programs, and supporting encore careers can benefit older individuals and contribute to economic growth and innovation.

To ensure a better future with extended lifespans, we must base our actions on the principles of environmental sustainability. Adopting sustainable practices, reducing carbon footprints, and preserving natural resources ensure that future generations can also enjoy a high quality of life.

Designing cities and urban spaces with an emphasis on pedestrian mobility, green spaces, and age-friendly infrastructure benefits older adults and promotes environmental sustainability. Access to nature, public transportation, and pedestrian-friendly environments encourages physical activity, reduces pollution, and creates livable communities.

Embracing a circular economy, which focuses on minimizing waste, promoting recycling, and reducing resource consumption, is essential for long-term sustainability. Encouraging responsible consumption, promoting renewable energy sources, and developing eco-friendly technologies contribute to a better future while promoting a longer lifespan.

A better future with a longer lifespan requires a multidimensional approach that addresses health and well-being, social dynamics, economic considerations, and environmental sustainability. By prioritizing preventive healthcare, fostering intergenerational connections, developing age-inclusive policies, and embracing sustainability, societies can create a future that values longevity and ensures a high quality of life for individuals of all ages. Through collective efforts and forward-thinking strategies, a future can be shaped where longer lifespans are accompanied by improvements in health, well-being, social cohesion, economic prosperity, and environmental stewardship.

As we close the final pages of this journey, we are filled with immense gratitude for those who have contributed to this book. Nineteen authors contributed to this English edition of 'The Korean Centenarian Study.' As mentioned in the preface, this book includes some content from the authors' 2021 publication, '*Korean centenarians: 20 years of change*' but most of it was newly written. The authors thank Dr. Kwang-Seog Kim, Mr. Sang Hyup Park, and Ms. Hwa Joung Yun from Chonnam National University Press for their diligent efforts in publishing this book. We also thank Dr. Hyun-Sook Lee from the Advanced Institute for Aging Science (AIAS) of Chonnam National University for her meticulous work in collecting and editing the manuscript. Additionally, we appreciate the cooperation and support of the researchers at the AIAS and the Korean Centenarian Study Group of Chonnam National University Hospital, Gwangju, Republic of Korea.